Management of acute and chronic neck pain

An evidence-based approach

Pain Research and Clinical Management

Other volumes in this series:

PAIN RESEARCH AND
CLINICAL MANAGEMENT

Management of acute and chronic neck pain

An evidence-based approach

Nikolai Bogduk BSc(Med) MB BS MD PhD
DSc Dip Anat Dip Pain Med FAFRM FAFMM
FFPM(ANZCA)
Conjoint Professor of Pain Medicine
University of Newcastle
Department of Clinical Research
Royal Newcastle Hospital
Newcastle New South Wales Australia

Brian McGuirk MB BS DPH FAFOM FAFMM
Senior Staff Specialist in Musculoskeletal Occupational Medicine
Hunter New England Area Health Service
Department of Clinical Research
Royal Newcastle Hospital
Newcastle New South Wales Australia

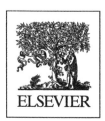

ELSEVIER

EDINBURGH LONDON NEW YORK OXFORD PHILADELPHIA ST LOUIS SYDNEY TORONTO 2006

ELSEVIER

© 2006, Elsevier BV. All rights reserved.

First published 2006

ISBN-10: 0 444 50846 5
ISBN-13: 978-0-444-50846-1

British Library Cataloguing in Publication Data
A catalogue record for this book is available from the British Library

Library of Congress Cataloging in Publication Data
A catalog record for this book is available from the Library of Congress

Notice
Knowledge and best practice in this field are constantly changing. As new research and experience broaden our knowledge, changes in practice, treatment and drug therapy may become necessary or appropriate. Readers are advised to check the most current information provided (i) on procedures featured or (ii) by the manufacturer of each product to be administered, to verify the recommended dose or formula, the method and duration of administration, and contraindications. It is the responsibility of the practitioner, relying on their own experience and knowledge of the patient, to make diagnoses, to determine dosages and the best treatment for each individual patient, and to take all appropriate safety precautions. To the fullest extent of the law, neither the Publisher nor the Authors assume any liability for any injury and/or damage to persons or property arising out or related to any use of the material contained in this book.

The Publisher

For Elsevier:

Commissioning Editor: Timothy Horne
Development Editor: Hannah Kenner
Project Manager: Gail Wright
Designer: Stewart Larking

Printed and bound in the United Kingdom
Transferred to Digital Print 2010

The publisher's policy is to use paper manufactured from sustainable forests

Preface

Since the advent of evidence-based medicine it has become fashionable for experts to compose systematic reviews of various treatments for musculo-skeletal pain. Neck pain has been no exception. These reviews serve a worth-while academic purpose. They concentrate into one resource all the leading studies of particular interventions. Systematic reviews, however, come at a price. Typically they are burdened with details of methodology and by the style of presentation that has become conventional for this type of publication. Although systematic reviews analyze the available evidence, all too often, they fail to provide guidelines to practitioners as to what to do in the face of that evidence.

In this text, we have taken a more utilitarian approach. We have dispensed with the formalities of methodology. We avoid the technical aspects of scoring and ranking studies for methodological rigor and quality. Nevertheless, we rely on the available evidence, but we focus on what the evidence means for practitioners, and on what practitioners can and should do, in the light of that evidence.

In composing the text, we have not been partisan. We do not represent any particular, traditional, craft group or specialty. We do not owe allegiance to any established way of doing things. Our only allegiance is to the evidence. In that regard, the definition of evidence-based medicine that we follow can be encapsulated by the acronym: RVE.

> **R** Reliability
> **V** Validity
> **E** Efficacy

We see evidence-based medicine as practice that aspires to use procedures that are reliable and valid, and treatments that are known to be effective; but perhaps more decisively, evidence-based medicine avoids practices that lack reliability, validity, or efficacy.

It is by avoiding unreliable, invalid, and ineffective practices that we distance ourselves from many established groups and specialties. Indeed, some readers might find our depiction of the evidence alienating, for research into neck pain has succeeded more often in showing what does not work than showing what does work. It transpires that much of what was taught and learned in the past is wrong.

On less contentious matters, we defer to available systematic reviews for their conclusions. On matters where practices or beliefs are well entrenched but which the evidence refutes, we not only refer to systematic reviews but also examine the source literature closely, in order to demonstrate to readers how weak the evidence is.

In the body of the text, we avoid pursuing matters of statistical argument. However, we do cite statistics, when available, to reinforce our conclusions quantitatively. For those unfamiliar with statistical jargon, in Part 6 we have provided an explanation of the terms that we use.

Our objective is to relate to practitioners what they should understand about neck pain, and how they should manage it. To this end we have divided the text into five parts.

Part 1 deals with matters of general principle: what might be portrayed as the "theory" of neck pain. That part covers the definition of neck pain, so that there is no confusion about the entity in question. It provides a background to the causes of neck pain and its risk factors, for these are seminal to understanding why and how neck pain arises; and they provide a basis for its treatment.

Part 2 deals with acute neck pain. It contains chapters that reflect, in logical and chronological order, what a practitioner might think and do when faced with a patient with acute neck pain.

The chapter on Natural History reflects what the practitioner should expect will happen to the patient's complaint, and arms the practitioner with what they can explain to the patient. Since data on natural history is evidence, explaining natural history becomes as much evidence-based practice as any other intervention.

During an actual consultation the practitioner is likely to take a history and perform a physical examination. The respective chapters on these topics provide a synopsis of the contemporary evidence on History and on Physical Examination as they pertain to neck pain. They explain what should be done and what is superfluous.

The practitioner might be tempted to order investigations. The chapters on Imaging and on Electrophysiological Tests explain why these are not necessary, and why they should be avoided.

The final chapters of this part outline an algorithm for the management of acute neck pain and provide the evidence that justifies what has been included and what has been excluded.

Part 3 addresses persistent or chronic neck pain. The chapters describe what is known about its causes and how these predicate its investigation and treatment.

A management algorithm is developed and defended by reference to the available evidence.

Part 4 provides a synopsis of the mechanisms of whiplash. In earlier chapters, whiplash is mentioned as one of the leading causes of neck pain, but in the context of assessment and management a detailed consideration of the mechanisms of whiplash is not immediately material. However, Part 4 is not an afterthought. The mechanisms of whiplash have been deliberately placed last in the text so as not to interfere with the momentum of the earlier sections, which are devoted to practical, clinical themes.

Part 5 deals with the particular entity of cervicogenic headache. This entity has been controversial for a variety of reasons, but fundamentally represents no more than neck pain referred to the head. It is as much an extension of neck pain as part of the differential diagnosis of headache.

Some of the chapters in these sections are deliberately detailed. Some readers might care not to be overwhelmed or oppressed by such detail. In order, nevertheless, to retain these readers, certain chapters have been written in abridged form. The abridged chapters provide the essential message about the forthcoming topic, with a clinically applied focus. Readers who want to avoid extended reading can go straight to these chapters. After doing so, if they remain unsatisfied, they can consult the succeeding chapters, in which the evidence is analyzed and presented in academic detail.

Accordingly, the short course through this book would be:

Chapter 1, to understand the definition of neck pain;

Chapter 2, to understand what are not causes of neck pain;

Chapter 4, to appreciate the favorable natural history;

Chapter 5, to discover how to rule out serious causes;

Chapter 7, to understand why imaging is not warranted;

Chapter 9, to learn how to manage acute neck pain;

Chapter 14, to learn how to assess patients with chronic neck pain;

Chapter 15, for the evidence on the treatment of chronic neck pain;

Chapter 16, for a summary of the mechanisms of whiplash and its symptoms;

Chapter 20, for a summary of cervicogenic headache.

Part 6 constitutes the explanations of statistical terms used in the clinical chapters of the text.

Contents

1 General principles

1 Definition

KEY POINTS

- Neck pain is pain perceived anywhere in the posterior region of the cervical spine, from the superior nuchal line to the first thoracic spinous process.

- Neck pain is not synonymous with cervical radicular pain. The two entities should be distinguished and considered separately.

- Neck pain may be referred to the head, upper limb girdle, and chest wall;

but

- somatic referred pain is not synonymous with cervical radicular pain;

- acute neck pain is neck pain that has been present for less than 3 months;

- chronic neck pain is neck pain that has been present for longer than 3 months.

CERVICAL SPINAL PAIN

In its *Classification of Chronic Pain,*[1] the International Association for the Study of Pain does not define "neck pain"; rather, it offers the following definition of *cervical spinal pain*:

> *pain perceived as arising from anywhere within the region bounded superiorly by the superior nuchal line, inferiorly by an imaginary transverse line through the tip of the first thoracic spinous process, and laterally by sagittal planes tangential to the lateral borders of the neck.*[1]

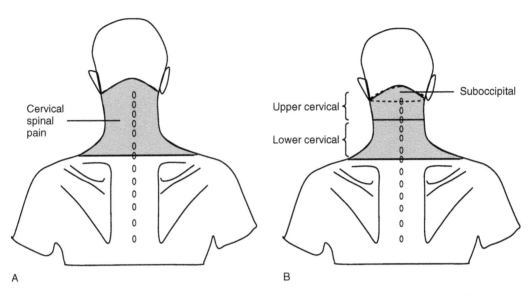

Figure 1.1 The topographical definition of neck pain. (A) Neck pain is posterior cervical spinal pain, which is pain anywhere between the superior nuchal line and a line through the T1 spinous process. (B) Neck pain can be divided into upper cervical and lower cervical spinal pain, either side of a transverse line through C4. Suboccipital pain is pain immediately below the superior nuchal line.

Implicit in this definition is that cervical spinal pain is perceived posteriorly (Figure 1.1A). This is consistent with how most patients use the term "neck pain". When they indicate neck pain they point to the back of the cervical spine. Pain to the front of the cervical spine would be described as pain in the throat, but not as neck pain. The present text follows this naming convention and in it neck pain is synonymous with cervical spinal pain.

The *Classification of Chronic Pain*[1] allows for a subdivision of cervical spinal pain (and therefore, neck pain) into *upper cervical spinal pain* and *lower cervical spinal pain*, above or below an imaginary transverse line that divides the cervical spinal region into equal halves (Figure 1.1B). It also allows for *suboccipital pain*, which is defined as pain located between the superior nuchal line and an imaginary transverse line passing through the tip of the second cervical spinous process.

Suboccipital pain invites a consideration of headache, and cervicogenic headache in particular. Because that topic involves a separate body of literature, it is addressed separately in Part 5.

Although some practitioners might recognize an entity called anterior neck pain, the very need to use the modifier "anterior" is evidence that they are referring to a special, if not unusual, entity, and one that is not adequately described by the term "neck pain" alone. Anterior neck pain has not been defined by an international authority, but could be defined as pain *ostensibly* stemming from the cervical spine but perceived

anteriorly in the region of the throat. Practitioners wishing to recognize such an entity would be obliged to show that the pain does, in fact, stem from the cervical spine and does not arise from the anterior cervical viscera.

RADICULAR PAIN

Quite emphatically, neck pain is not synonymous with cervical radicular pain or brachialgia. Although it may occur in association with neck pain, cervical radicular pain is pain *perceived in the upper limb*. Its causes are different from those of neck pain, and the evidence-base for its diagnosis and management is distinctly different. If for no other reason, neck pain and cervical radicular pain should be discussed and taught as separate entities, lest practitioners and students confuse the two and end up applying investigations and treatments that might be appropriate for radicular pain but which are totally inappropriate for neck pain. The topic of cervical radicular pain has been addressed in detail elsewhere.[2,3,4] Making the distinction between radicular pain and neck pain is addressed in Chapter 5.

SOMATIC REFERRED PAIN

Referred pain is pain perceived in a region innervated by nerves other than those that innervate the source of the pain.[5] Its mechanism is believed to be convergence on common neurons in the central nervous system of afferent impulses from the two regions concerned.

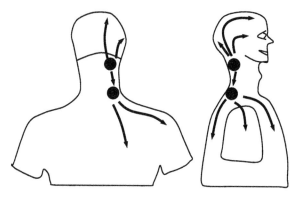

Figure 1.2 Directions in which cervical spinal pain can be referred. Upper cervical pain can be referred to the occiput, frontal region, and orbit, as well as caudally into the neck. Lower cervical pain can be referred to the shoulder, the scapular region, or the anterior chest wall.

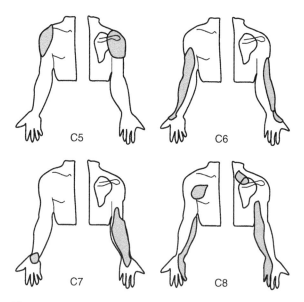

Figure 1.3 Patterns of referred pain evoked from the interspinous muscles at the segments indicated. Based on Kellgren.[6] The pain is perceived distally, away from the cervical spine, into the upper limb.

From sources in the cervical spine, pain can be referred to various regions: the head, the upper limb, the interscapular region, and the anterior chest wall (Figure 1.2). As a rule, patterns of referral are a function of the *segmental* location of the primary source of pain. From upper cervical segments, pain is typically referred to the head. From lower cervical segments it can be referred into the anterior chest wall, interscapular region, or upper limb. The basis for these rules lies in several experimental studies using normal volunteers and in certain clinical studies.

The earliest studies of somatic referred pain involved stimulating the cervical interspinous spaces of normal volunteers with painful injections of hypertonic saline.[6,7] Each such injection was associated with a particular pattern of distribution of referred pain (Figure 1.3). These studies indicated that cervical pain could be referred into distal regions of the upper limb.

Subsequent studies have not confirmed this type of distribution when other structures in the cervical spine have been stimulated; nor has it been verified in patients suffering from neck pain and pain in the upper limb. In normal volunteers[8] and in volunteer patients,[9] noxious stimulation of the cervical zygapophysial joints produces patterns of pain that spread only into the upper limb girdle and, at most, into the proximal arm (Figure 1.4). In clinical studies,[10,11,12] pain in these distributions has been relieved by anesthetizing cervical zygapophysial joints, but no studies have reported relief of pain in the distal arm, forearm, or hand following anesthetization of cervical zygapophysial joints.

From cervical intervertebral discs,[13,14] patterns of referred pain have been observed similar to those produced by the zygapophysial joints (Figure 1.4). This indicates that it is not the structure that is associated with

a typical pattern of referred pain, but its segmental location and innervation. All structures innervated by the same segmental nerves can produce referred pain in a territory that is relatively specific for those segments.

There have been no formal studies in normal volunteers of referred pain to the anterior chest wall.

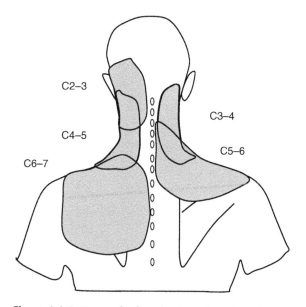

Figure 1.4 Patterns of referred pain evoked from the cervical zygapophysial joints and intervertebral discs. Based on Dwyer et al.,[8] Schellhas et al.,[13] and Grubb and Kelly.[14]

However, modern studies have noted that some patients can have pain in the chest wall that arises in the lower cervical intervertebral discs.[14]

Headache can be produced by experimental noxious stimulation of the C2–3 zygapophysial joints,[8] the lateral atlanto-axial joints,[15] and the atlanto-occipital joints.[15] Conspicuously, these joints are innervated by the C3, C2, and C1 spinal nerves, respectively.[16,17] It is these segments that are most often responsible for referred pain to the head. Clinical studies have confirmed that the C2–3 zygapophysial joints[18] and the lateral atlanto-axial joints[19] can be sources of headache. It is uncommon for headaches to be referred from segments below C3.[20]

Somatic referred pain should not be confused with radicular pain. The two are not synonymous: their causes differ, as do their mechanisms. However, although it is necessary to distinguish between the two, it is not always easy to do so clinically. Guidelines for this purpose are provided in Chapter 5.

ACUTE AND CHRONIC

By convention, the International Association for the Study of Pain uses a temporal basis for defining, and distinguishing, acute and chronic pain. For pain not due to cancer, it accepts 3 months as a convenient point of division. Thus, acute pain is pain that has been present for less than 3 months while pain lasting longer than 3 months constitutes chronic pain.

In the context of neck pain, it has not been commonplace for investigators to distinguish subacute pain (i.e. pain for less than 3 months but more than 7 weeks), as it has been in the context of low back pain. Nor have there been any studies of treatment that have identified a difference in response to the same intervention between patients with subacute neck pain and those with either acute or chronic neck pain. Therefore, in the present text, no such distinction is drawn. It seems practical to identify and distinguish only acute and chronic neck pain.

References

1. Merskey H, Bogduk N (eds). Classification of Chronic Pain. Descriptions of Chronic Pain Syndromes and Definitions of Pain Terms, 2nd edn. IASP Press, Seattle, 1994: 11.
2. Bogduk N. Medical Management of Acute Cervical Radicular Pain: An Evidence-Based Approach. Newcastle Bone and Joint Institute, Newcastle, 1999.
3. Bogduk N. Neck and arm pain. In: Aminoff MJ, Daroff RB (eds). Encyclopedia of the Neurological Sciences, Volume 3. Academic Press, Amsterdam, 2003: 390–398.
4. Bogduk N. Cervical pain. In: Ashbury AK, McKhann GM, McDonald WI, Goadsby PJ, MacArthur JC (eds). Disease of the Nervous system. Clinical Neuroscience and Therapeutic Principles. Cambridge University Press, Cambridge, 2002: 742–759.
5. Merskey H, Bogduk N (eds). Classification of Chronic Pain. Descriptions of Chronic pain Syndromes and Definitions of Pain Terms, 2nd edn. IASP Press, Seattle, 1994: 12.
6. Kellgren JH. On the distribution of pain arising from deep somatic structures with charts of segmental pain areas. Clin Sci 1939; 4: 35–46.
7. Feinstein B, Langton JBK, Jameson RM, Schiller F. Experiments on referred pain from deep somatic tissues. J Bone Joint Surg 1954; 36A: 981–997.
8. Dwyer A, Aprill C, Bogduk N. Cervical zygapophyseal joint pain patterns I: a study in normal volunteers. Spine 1990; 15: 453–457.
9. Fukui S, Ohseto K, Shiotani M, Ohno K, Karasawa H, Nagaauma Y, Yuda Y. Referred pain distribution of the cervical zygapophyseal joints and cervical dorsal rami. Pain 1996; 68: 79–83.
10. Bogduk N, Marsland A. The cervical zygapophysial joints as a source of neck pain. Spine 1988; 13: 610–617.
11. Barnsley L, Lord SM, Wallis BJ, Bogduk N. The prevalence of chronic cervical zygapophysial joint pain after whiplash. Spine 1995; 20: 20–26.
12. Lord S, Barnsley L, Wallis BJ, Bogduk N. Chronic cervical zygapophysial joint pain after whiplash: a placebo-controlled prevalence study. Spine 1996; 21: 1737–1745.
13. Schellhas KP, Smith MD, Gundry CR, Pollei SR. Cervical discogenic pain: prospective correlation of magnetic resonance imaging and discography in asymptomatic subjects and pain sufferers. Spine 1996; 21: 300–312.
14. Grubb JA, Kelly CK. Cervical discography: clinical implications from twelve years' experience. Spine 2000; 25: 1382–1389.
15. Dreyfuss P, Michaelsen M, Fletcher D. Atlanto-occipital and lateral atlanto-axial joint pain patterns. Spine 1994; 19: 1125–1131.
16. Bogduk N. The clinical anatomy of the cervical dorsal rami. Spine 1982; 7: 319–330.
17. Lazorthes G, Gaubert J. L'innervation des articulations interapophysaire vertebrales. Comptes Rendues de l'Association des Anatomistes 1956: 488–494.
18. Lord S, Barnsley L, Wallis B, Bogduk N. Third occipital nerve headache: a prevalence study. J Neurol Neurosurg Psychiatry 1994; 57: 1187–1190.
19. Aprill C, Axinn MJ, Bogduk N. Occipital headaches stemming from the lateral atlanto-axial (C1–2) joint. Cephalalgia 2002; 22: 15–22.
20. Lord SM, Bogduk N. The cervical synovial joints as sources of post-traumatic headache. J Musculoskeletal Pain 1996; 4: 81–94.

2

Sources and causes of neck pain

KEY POINTS

- Any of the innervated structures of the cervical spine can be a source of neck pain.

- Serious and identifiable causes of neck pain are rare.

- The cause or causes of common neck pain are not known.

- Cervical spondylosis is not a legitimate diagnosis of neck pain.

- Among the important but rare causes of neck pain are tumors, infections, fractures, and aneurysms of the vertebral or internal carotid arteries.

It is relevant here to distinguish between "source" and "cause," for the two terms can be confused or misrepresented. Furthermore, in some instances, although the cause of pain might not be found, its source might nevertheless be established.

The *source* of pain is the anatomical structure from which nociceptive activity is generated which, in turn, leads to the perception of pain. Sources of pain are, therefore, specified by naming the structure, without reference to the pathology responsible for the pain.

The *cause* of pain is the actual disorder or disease responsible for generating the nociceptive activity in the structure that is the source of pain. Causes of pain are specified in pathological terms.

In the context of neck pain, much is known about its possible sources, but little about actual sources. Similarly, although much is known about rare causes of neck pain, virtually nothing is known about common causes.

SOURCES

The possible sources of neck pain are dictated by the innervation of the cervical spine. In principle, any structure that receives a nerve supply may become a source of pain if it is affected by an appropriate disorder.

The innervated structures that are found throughout the cervical spine are: the zygapophysial joints and the posterior neck muscles;[1] the cervical intervertebral discs;[2,3,4] the vertebral bodies;[4] the anterior and posterior longitudinal ligaments;[2,4] the dura mater of the cervical spinal cord;[5,6] and the prevertebral muscles. At upper cervical levels, the innervated structures are: the atlanto-occipital and atlanto-axial joints;[7] and the transverse ligament.[5] To this list must be added the vertebral artery, for it is innervated by cervical nerves.[8,9] Similarly, the internal carotid artery presumably has a cervical innervation, although the source of this innervation has not been explicitly demonstrated.

(In the cervical spine interspinous ligaments are lacking and therefore these structures cannot be sources of neck pain. The ligamentum nuchae does not constitute a ligament; it is a raphe between the trapezius muscles, the rhomboid muscles, and the splenius muscles.[10] Its innervation, therefore, is accounted for by the innervation of these muscles.)

Notwithstanding this list of possible sources of neck pain, no data are available concerning the actual prevalence with which *acute neck pain* arises from muscles, joints, discs, ligaments, or the dura mater. Although various authorities may have their own views on this matter, explicit data are lacking. The main reason for this is that there are no reliable and valid ways of establishing an anatomical diagnosis that are suitable for use in patients with acute neck pain (Chapters 6 and 7). Some data are available for patients with *chronic neck pain*, and these are discussed in Chapters 12 and 13.

CAUSES

In chapters on neck pain, textbooks often list the possible causes of neck pain (Table 2.1), but they have typically done so without regard to the validity of the diagnosis and without regard to prevalence. Most of the conditions so listed are either rare or contentious, with little (or conflicting) evidence that they are, indeed, causes of neck pain.

Serious but rare causes

Certain conditions are recognizable and serious but rare causes of neck pain (Table 2.1). These include *tumors* of the vertebral column (both primary and secondary), *infections* of the bones, joints, or discs of the cervical spine, and meningitis of the cervical dura mater.

Tumors and infections are largely recognizable since they can be detected by medical imaging (Chapter 7). Difficulties obtain only when the lesions are early or small. Meningitis is readily suspected on clinical grounds (fever, neck stiffness, Kernig's sign) and confirmed by lumbar puncture. That these conditions are valid causes

of neck pain is based not on formal experimental data but on clinical experience, in that treating the conditions successfully results in resolution of the neck pain.

These conditions are serious because they pose an immediate threat to the patient's health. Tumors can continue to grow and threaten the spinal cord or the stability of the cervical vertebral column; or they can metastasize. Infections can spread systemically, and abscesses can threaten the spinal cord or the integrity of the vertebral column.

There have been no studies published indicating the prevalence of these conditions in primary care, nor are there any epidemiological data on their prevalence in secondary or tertiary care. Inferential data, however, indicate that they are quite rare in primary care. Two population studies of plain radiography of the cervical spine, each involving over 1000 patients, reported not detecting any serious disorder that was not otherwise suspected.[14,15] By inference, this zero prevalence of undiagnosed tumors or infections has an upper 95% confidence limit of 0.4%. Thus, it can confidently be deduced that *serious causes of neck pain have a prevalence substantially less than 0.4%*.

Most of the substantive literature on spinal osteomyelitis and epidural abscesses is generic, in that it pertains to these conditions across all regions of the spine.[16-21] Very little information is available concerning the features of these conditions when they affect just the neck.

A cervical *epidural abscess* can present with neck pain, prior to producing neurological signs. As a cause of neck pain, however, it is considered very rare. In most cases the history or physical examination suggests a reason for infection (such as surgery or injection in the cervical region) or reveals a distant source;[17,22-26] but some authorities consider that it can occur rarely in the absence of obvious predisposing factors or sources.[27] Interestingly, the one case report of so-called spontaneous epidural abscess[27] describes a patient in whom cultures were not diagnostic but who had all the clinical hallmarks of retropharyngeal tendonitis (see below). The two conditions, therefore, might mimic one another, when neck pain is the only presenting feature.

Spontaneous *epidural hematoma* is a condition that can develop with no apparent cause, or after a seemingly trivial event such as sneezing or straining, the most likely unifying event being an increase in spinal epidural pressure.[28] Once recognized, epidural hematoma is a neurosurgical emergency, the objective of which is to decompress the spinal cord. The definitive diagnosis is made by CT or MRI, and the indicative features are the onset of neurological signs.

The initial presenting feature of epidural hematoma may simply be neck pain. Case reports describing cervical

Table 2.1 Causes of neck pain as listed in three major textbooks of rheumatology,[11,12,13] showing also the extent to which these sources agree

Causes	Nakano[11]	Hardin and Halla[12]	Binder[13]
Serious but rare			
Vertebral tumors	++	++	++
Discitis	++	++	00
Septic arthritis	++	++	00
Osteomyelitis	++	++	++
Meningitis	++	++	00
Epidural abscess	00	00	00
Epidural hematoma	00	00	00
Valid but rare or unusual			
Rheumatoid arthritis	++	++	++
Ankylosing spondylitis	++	++	00
Crystal arthropathies including gout	++	++	++
Polymyalgia rheumatica	00	++	++
Longus colli tendonitis	00	++	00
Fractures	00	++	00
Synovial cyst	00	++	00
Miscellaneous			
Torticollis	++	++	++
Detectable but of questionable validity			
Diffuse idiopathic skeletal hyperostosis	++	++	++
Ossification of the posterior longitudinal ligament	00	00	++
Paget's disease	++	++	++
Spondylosis/degenerative disease	++	++	++
Osteoarthritis	++	00	00
Neurological			
Thoracic outlet syndrome	++	++	++
Spinal cord tumors	++	00	00
Nerve injuries	++	00	00
Myelopathy	00	00	++
Radiculopathy	00	00	++

Continued

Table 2.1 Causes of neck pain as listed in three major textbooks of rheumatology,[11,12,13] showing also the extent to which these sources agree—cont'd

Causes	Nakano[11]	Hardin and Halla[12]	Binder[13]
Spurious or vague			
Soft-tissue injuries	00	++	00
Whiplash	00	00	++
Cervical strain	++	00	00
Psychogenic	00	00	++
Postural disorders	++	00	++
Fibrositis, myofascial pain	++	++	++
Hyoid bone syndrome	00	++	00
Sternocleidomastoid tendonitis	++	00	00
Fibromyalgia	00	++	00

+: mentioned by the text cited
0: not mentioned by the text cited

epidural hematoma typically commence with a history of undiagnosed neck pain.[28,29] Notwithstanding, the possibility of epidural hematoma is not a pretext for implementing investigations. The pre-test probability of epidural hematoma is so low that the pre-emptive use of advanced imaging such as CT or MRI is extremely wasteful. Investigations should be reserved until there is an indication of the onset of neurological features. Motor and sensory deficits develop, usually within hours of the onset of pain.[28,30,31] Patients presenting with neck pain should be warned to report immediately the onset of any new clinical features, at which time the instigation of investigations can be reconsidered.

One model of the pathology of epidural hematoma is that it arises as a result of bursting of an epidural vein.[29,30] Another model invokes rupture of a spinal artery.[29,30] Given these models, anticoagulant therapy,[32,33,34] including excessive consumption of garlic,[35] is a risk factor for spontaneous epidural hematoma.

Valid but rare or unusual causes

Certain conditions can be considered valid causes of pain when recognized in patients with neck pain (Table 2.1). They are valid on the grounds that they are accepted causes of pain when encountered elsewhere in the body. Some are not necessarily rare conditions but are systemic disorders that rarely affect just the neck. Others are rare in their own right.

By definition, *rheumatoid arthritis* is a polyarticular disease. The upper cervical spine is one area of the body that can be affected, but when rheumatoid arthritis affects the neck it does so in patients with disease of the appendicular joints, and in whom the diagnosis is already evident. Only rarely does rheumatoid arthritis present as neck pain with no peripheral manifestations.[36] Rheumatoid arthritis poses a potential serious threat to the spinal cord when it affects the C1–2 segment, but even then the prognosis is favorable.[37]

Similar comments apply to *ankylosing spondylitis*. Although ankylosing spondylitis can affect the cervical spine, it does so typically late in the evolution of the disease, and in patients in whom the diagnosis is already evident on the basis of sacroiliac and other joint involvement. Some 10% of patients with ankylosing spondylitis may present with neck pain,[38] but the rarity of ankylosing spondylitis renders it an uncommon cause of neck pain.

Involvement of the cervical spine is uncommon in *Reiter's syndrome*.[12] When it does occur, it seems to have a predilection for the C1–2 segment and the craniocervical junction.[39,40] *Psoriatic arthritis* can have a pattern of joint involvement similar to that of rheumatoid arthritis or that of ankylosing spondylitis.[12] As such, it is a systemic condition that can involve the neck, but is a rare cause of neck pain alone.

Gout typically has a predilection for joints of the appendicular skeleton, and although it can affect the spine, it does so rarely.[12] Similarly, various other crystal arthropathies can affect the cervical spine, but since they are rare conditions in their own right, they are rare causes of neck pain.

Like rheumatoid arthritis, *polymyalgia rheumatica* is a systemic disorder. Although the neck can be one area of the body that is involved, this condition, by definition, does not affect just the neck;[13,41] and so cannot be considered a legitimate differential diagnosis of neck pain.

Longus colli tendonitis is a misnomer for a condition that lacks a suitably accurate name. The condition is also known as *retropharyngeal tendonitis*;[42,43,44] however, it involves more than just the tendons of the prevertebral muscles. It involves inflammation and edema of the upper portions of the longus colli (not just its tendons) from the level of C1 to C4 and even as far caudally as C6.[42,43,44] It has been reported in occasional case reports, and is considered a rare condition. One estimate places the incidence at about 1 per 400 000 population per year.[42] The inflammation is often associated with calcification opposite the C2 vertebra,[42-48] but calcification appears to be an epiphenomenon unrelated to the pain, for chronic calcification at the same site can be painless.[49] Inflammation of the longus colli or prevertebral-retropharyngeal space seems to be the cardinal correlate with pain.

Fractures are an accepted cause of pain, although not all fractures are necessarily painful. As causes of neck pain, however, fractures are rare or unusual. Like tumors, unsuspected fractures proved to have zero prevalence in large population surveys,[14,15] which places their prevalence at less than 0.4%. Even among patients presenting to emergency rooms with suspected or possible cervical trauma, fractures are uncommon (Table 2.2). A prevalence figure of 3.5% ($\pm$ 0.5%) would be representative.

Torticollis

Although listed as a cause of neck pain, torticollis is a distinctive entity in its own right. The diagnosis is established not by the presence of neck pain but by the characteristic rotatory deformity with which the patient presents, and from which the condition gets its name. By definition, however, torticollis is not a differential diagnosis of neck pain, for without the deformity the patient cannot have torticollis. Reciprocally, the differential diagnosis of torticollis in adults includes mechanical cervical causes such as extrapment of a meniscoid in a cervical zygapophysial joint,[59] atlanto-axial subluxation,[60-64] or vertebral osteomyelitis,[65] but also includes non-cervical causes that may be of a more pernicious nature, such as a basal ganglion disorder or phenothiazine toxicity.

Detectable but questionable disorders

Diffuse idiopathic skeletal hyperostosis is a condition vividly demonstrable on radiographs of affected regions of the spine. Although listed as a cause of neck pain,

Table 2.2 The prevalence of fractures on plain films of the cervical spine in patients with putative neck injuries. Based on Roberge et al.[53]

Size of sample	Prevalence	Source
107	5%	50
233	10%	51
351	2%	52
467	1.7%	53
446	2%	54
860	2.8%	55
974	2.8%	56
1331	4.6%	57
1823	3.5%	58
Weighted mean	**3.5%**	

it is often asymptomatic.[12,13] When symptomatic, it causes stiffness and dysphagia rather than neck pain.[12,13] Similarly, ossification of the posterior longitudinal ligament can be asymptomatic.[12,13] Rather than neck pain, this condition is more likely to present with myelopathy.[12,13]

Paget's disease is, as a general rule, an accepted cause of pain in the body regions affected. Technically, therefore, it is an acceptable cause of neck pain if detected in the cervical spine. However, one large survey found that Paget's disease is often painless, and that patients with cervical spine involvement had no pain complaints referable to that region.[66] This finding gives cause to doubt that Paget's disease is ever a cause of neck pain. When diagnosed radiologically, Paget's disease in the cervical spine may be no more than an incidental finding.

Although listed as a cause of neck pain, synovial cysts in the cervical spine do not cause neck pain. All case reports of this rare condition indicate that cysts cause myelopathy or radiculopathy, by compressing the spinal cord or a spinal nerve.[67,68,69] Neither of these conditions constitutes neck pain.

Spondylosis

Purists might prefer to distinguish spondylosis from osteoarthritis of the cervical spine. In that event, spondylosis is a disorder affecting the vertebral bodies and intervertebral discs, and is characterized essentially by the presence of osteophytes around the vertebral margins. In contrast, osteoarthritis is a disorder of the synovial joints of the cervical spine: the zygapophysial joints and the atlanto-axial joints. Yet it, too, is characterized by osteophytes, as well as joint narrowing, and subchondral sclerosis. When not distinguished, these two conditions collectively are referred to as degenerative joint disease.

Spondylosis and osteoarthrosis, or degenerative joint disease, are regularly listed as causes of neck pain, but the evidence expressly refutes this association. Individual radiographic features of cervical spondylosis occur with increasing frequency with increasing age in asymptomatic individuals[70,71] (Tables 2.3 and 2.4). This indicates that these features are age-related changes. Age changes most commonly affect the C5–6 and C6–7 segments, with those segments above and below these levels being progressively less commonly affected (Table 2.5).

In some studies cervical spondylosis occurs slightly more commonly in symptomatic individuals than in asymptomatic individuals,[14,72] but the odds ratios for disc degeneration or osteoarthrosis as predictors of neck pain are only 1.1 and 0.97 respectively for women,

and 1.7 and 1.8 for men.[72] In other studies, the prevalence of disc degeneration at individual segments of the neck is not significantly different between symptomatic patients and asymptomatic controls.[73] Indeed, uncovertebral osteophytes and osteoarthrosis were found to be less prevalent in symptomatic individuals.[73]

Neurological causes

Neurological disorders are not legitimate differential diagnoses of neck pain, for their cardinal presenting feature is not neck pain but loss of neurological function, usually elsewhere, other than in the neck. Cervical radiculopathy and thoracic outlet syndrome are manifest by sensory and motor deficits in the upper limb. Cervical myelopathy is characterized by loss of function in the lower limbs. Spinal cord tumors may present with loss of function in either the upper or the lower limbs, depending on the location of the tumor.

Although these conditions may be associated with neck pain, it is the loss of neurological function that provides the diagnosis. Conversely, in the absence of

Table 2.3 The number of asymptomatic subjects exhibiting features of spondylosis by gender and age. Based on Gore et al.[70]

| Feature | Men by age group (N = 20 in each group) | | | | |
	20–25	30–35	40–45	50–55	60–65
Narrowing	0	1	4	13	15
Sclerosis	0	1	1	10	13
Anterior osteophytes	1	5	7	16	19
Posterior osteophytes	0	1	4	10	14
Any of the above	1	5	7	16	19
Women by age group (N = 20 in each group)					
Narrowing	0	2	6	9	13
Sclerosis	0	0	5	7	6
Anterior osteophytes	0	3	6	13	11
Posterior osteophytes	0	1	5	8	12
Any of the above	0	4	7	14	14
Men and women by age group (N = 40 in each group)					
Narrowing	0	1	4	13	15
Sclerosis	0	1	1	10	13
Anterior osteophytes	1	5	7	16	19
Posterior osteophytes	0	1	4	10	14
Any of the above	1	5	7	16	19

Table 2.4 The prevalence of radiological features of the cervical spine in asymptomatic individuals. Based on Elias[71]

| Feature | Number of subjects by age | | | |
	<30	30–40	40–50	>50
Normal	24	18	18	2
Osteophytes	0	3	7	14
Narrowing of disc space	0	0	7	18
Sclerosis of articular surface	0	0	0	7
Osteoporosis	0	0	0	4
Calcification of anterior ligament	0	0	0	4
Loss of lordosis	0	0	0	4
Number of patients	24	21	32	25
Males:females	5:19	7:14	20:12	18:7

neurological symptoms or signs, there are no grounds for suspecting these conditions in the differential diagnosis of neck pain.

There are, however, neurological disorders other than radiculopathy or myelopathy that can present with neck pain but no neurological signs, or signs that might be overlooked. These conditions are rare and have been described only in case reports.

Injuries to peripheral nerves of the shoulder girdle, such as the long thoracic nerve and the spinal accessory nerve, may not be readily apparent because they do not cause sensory problems, and patients may not be immediately aware of their motor deficits. Pain occurs not because of a cervical lesion but as a result of *neuromas* developing on the proximal stump of the severed nerve and affecting deep sensory afferents.[74] Since these afferents relay to cervical segments, the pain of the neuroma will be perceived as cervical pain.

One case report records an unusual cause of a particular type of neck pain.[75] The patient suffered paroxysmal pain in the region of the trapezius muscle. The cause was found to be irritation of the dorsal root entry zone of the sensory roots of the spinal accessory nerve by an aberrant vertebral artery.

Another case report describes two patients who presented with neck pain.[76] One was subsequently found to have a subarachnoid hemorrhage, the other a cerebral glioblastoma multiforme. The mechanism of pain was not discussed in the report, but these cases probably constitute examples of dural irritation—by blood in the first case and by a space-occupying lesion in the second. One would expect such lesions to produce headache, but since the tentorium cerebelli is innervated by cervical nerves, referral of pain to the neck is possible.

Spurious conditions

Certain terms proffered as diagnoses of neck pain, and listed as such by textbooks, do not constitute legitimate diagnoses. These include: soft-tissue injuries, whiplash, cervical strain, and psychogenic pain. "Soft-tissue injury"

Table 2.5 The prevalence (%) of age-changes by segmental level in 160 asymptomatic individuals. Based on Fridenberg and Miller[73]

| Feature | Segmental level | | | | | |
	C2–3	C3–4	C4–5	C5–6	C6–7	C7–T1
Disc degeneration		7	13	30	26	3
Uncovertebral osteophytes	3	13	24	30	31	3
Foraminal encroachment	1	11	14	23	21	1
Zygapophysial osteoarthrosis	2	6	7	6	2	

means no more than neck pain in the absence of a fracture,[77] the nature of the "injury" and its location, not being specified. "Whiplash" is a descriptor that pertains to the alleged etiology of the pain, not to its cause. "Cervical strain" is an inference, but does not specify the nature of the lesion or its location. "Psychogenic pain" lacks diagnostic criteria, and is an inference invoked when no other diagnosis is recognized.

Although some authorities attribute neck pain to postural abnormalities, this label lacks both reliability and validity (Chapter 6). Similarly, fibrositis and myofascial pain lack reliability and validity in the context of neck pain (Chapter 6). Tendonitis of the sternocleidomastoid or longus colli is an entity that lacks valid diagnostic criteria.

Fibromyalgia is, by definition, a disorder that must affect multiple regions of the body.[78] Although the neck may be one of these regions, the patient must have pain in other regions. Therefore, fibromyalgia is not a differential diagnosis that can be applied to a patient who presents with neck pain alone.

Hyoid bone syndrome is a contentious entity. It is said to be characterized by tenderness over the greater horn of the hyoid bone; and the diagnostic criterion is complete relief of pain upon anesthetization of this region.[79] However, no controlled studies have tested the validity of this criterion, and the prevalence of this condition is not known.

Vascular disorders

Overlooked by contemporary textbooks is the importance of vascular disorders in the diagnosis of neck pain. Although headache is the most common presenting feature of internal carotid artery dissection, neck pain has been the sole presenting feature in some 6% of cases.[80,81] In 17% of patients, headache may occur in combination with neck pain.[81] Neck pain has been the initial presenting feature in 50–90% of patients with vertebral artery dissection, but is usually also accompanied by headache, typically in the occipital region although not exclusively so.[80,82] Although the typical features of dissecting aneurysms of the aorta are chest pain and cardiovascular distress, neck pain has been reported as the presenting feature in some 6% of cases.[83,84]

Whiplash

Neck pain attributed to an injury sustained in a motor vehicle accident is an entity distinguished not by any unique cause but by the controversies concerning its cause and interpretation. The natural history of this complaint is such that the vast majority of patients recover (Chapter 4), which suggests that most patients sustain no substantive or lasting injury to their neck.

Perhaps they suffer a minor muscle sprain, or simply jarring of their neck. However, a minority of patients do develop chronic pain, and for these patients modern biomechanics studies have demonstrated a plausible mechanism of injury.[77] The possible causes of pain in these patients are considered in Chapter 12.

With respect to acute neck pain, whiplash poses similar problems to those associated with neck pain not due to whiplash. In most cases, a patho-anatomic diagnosis will not be evident, but like neck pain in general, neck pain after whiplash can sometimes be caused by certain serious injuries.

Fractures due to whiplash are so uncommon as to be rare. In one study of 283 patients with acute neck pain after whiplash, no fractures were found on plain radiography.[85] Assuming 0% to be the lower 95% confidence limit of the true prevalence, this result implies a prevalence of less than 1.3%. In a large prospective study of cervical spine radiography involving 8924 patients, 2788 had a history of a rear-end motor vehicle collision.[86] Of these, only two were found to have a fracture, placing the prevalence of fracture due to whiplash at 0.07%.

Such fractures as have been attributed to whiplash have been reported only in case studies or small descriptive series. These fractures may be difficult to detect on conventional investigations, and special attention needs to be paid to their possibility if they are to be detected (see Chapter 7). The majority involve the upper cervical spine, and include fractures of the odontoid process,[87,88] the laminae and articular processes of C2,[87,88,89] and the occipital condyles.[90] Others include fractures of the lower cervical spinous processes.[91]

Various lesions can affect the prevertebral region of the neck and compromise the respiratory tract or puncture the esophagus. These include prevertebral hematoma, either in isolation[92] or in association with an avulsion fracture of an anterior osteophyte.[93] Prominent anterior osteophytes can puncture the esophagus when the neck is forcefully extended.[94]

Vascular lesions can affect either the vertebral artery or the internal carotid artery. Either vessel can sustain a dissecting aneurysm after whiplash.[95,96] The vertebral artery can be injured in isolation or in association with a fracture of the second cervical vertebra adjacent to the artery.[97] Injury to the cervical portion (third part) of the vertebral artery can lead to thrombosis of the basilar artery.[98] The internal carotid artery can be strangulated by the hypoglossal nerve.[99]

SYNTHESIS

If neurological disorders, systemic disorders, and conditions of questionable validity are censored from traditional lists of the causes of neck pain, an interesting dichotomy arises (Table 2.6). At one extreme lie the detectable, serious, but rare conditions. At the other extreme, the common causes of neck pain are either spurious or unknown.

When a patho-anatomic diagnosis of neck pain cannot be made, the International Association for the Study of Pain (IASP) recommended that the term *cervical spinal pain of unknown origin* be applied.[100] Although cumbersome, this term honestly reflects the situation. The patient has pain ostensibly stemming from the cervical spine, but a specific diagnosis is lacking.

The IASP also recommended "acceleration-deceleration injury" as the preferred synonym for whiplash,[100] and recognized this entity as applying to neck pain with a distinctive etiology. This label does not presuppose any particular cause of pain (indeed, if any). It only recognizes neck pain with a particular attributed cause. It is, however, a clumsier expression than "whiplash," and has not succeeded in replacing the more colloquial appellation in the literature.

Otherwise, the IASP admitted entities such as cervical muscle sprain, and segmental dysfunction, but in doing so set strict diagnostic criteria that required valid and reliable diagnostic tests for these conditions. In the absence of such tests, these diagnoses cannot be made and are of theoretical interest only.

The IASP recognized the conditions of cervical zygapophysial joint pain and cervical discogenic pain, but stipulated diagnostic criteria that required invasive tests. For patients with acute neck pain these tests are inappropriate, but they may be of value in the assessment of patients with chronic neck pain. In that regard they are considered in Chapter 13.

For practical use, the Australian Acute Musculoskeletal Pain Guidelines[101] recommended two terms in the context of neck pain. For neck pain following, or attributed to, a motor vehicle accident, they accepted the term *whiplash-associated neck pain*. For neck pain with no known cause, they recommended *idiopathic neck pain*.

Table 2.6 A synopsis of the causes of neck pain

	Uncommon or rare	*Common*
Serious	Tumors	
	Infections	
	Crystal arthropathies	
	Fractures	
	Aneurysms	
	Neuromas	
Non-serious		Unknown
		Strain
		Whiplash

References

1. Bogduk N. The clinical anatomy of the cervical dorsal rami. Spine 1982; 7: 319–330.
2. Bogduk N, Windsor M, Inglis A. The innervation of the cervical intervertebral discs. Spine 1988; 13: 2–8.
3. Mendel T, Wink CS, Zimny ML. Neural elements in human cervical intervertebral discs. Spine 1992; 17: 132–135.
4. Groen GJ, Baljet B, Drukker J. Nerves and nerve plexuses of the human vertebral column. Am J Anat 1990; 188: 282–296.
5. Kimmel DL. Innervation of the spinal dura mater and dura mater of the posterior cranial fossa. Neurology 1960; 10: 800–809.
6. Groen GJ, Baljet B, Drukker J. The innervation of the spinal dura mater: anatomy and clinical implications. Acta Neurochir 1988; 92: 39–46.
7. Lazorthes G, Gaubert J. L'innervation des articulations interapophysaire vertebrales. Comptes Rendues de l'Association des Anatomistes 1956; 43: 488–494.
8. Kimmel DL. The cervical sympathetic rami and the vertebral plexus in the human foetus. J Comp Neurol 1959; 112: 141–161.
9. Bogduk N, Lambert G, Duckworth JW. The anatomy and physiology of the vertebral nerve in relation to cervical migraine. Cephalalgia 1981; 1: 11–24.
10. Mercer SR, Bogduk N. Clinical anatomy of ligamentum nuchae. Clin Anat 2003; 16: 484–493.
11. Nakano KK. Neck pain. In: Ruddy S, Harris ED, Sledge CB (eds). Kelley's Texbook of Rheumatology, 6th edn. WB Saunders, Philadelphia, 2001: 457–474.
12. Hardin JG, Halla JT. Cervical spine syndromes. In: Koopman WJ (ed). Arthritis and Allied Conditions: A Textbook of Rheumatology, 14th edn. Lippincott Williams & Wilkins, Philadelphia, 2001: 2009–2018.
13. Binder A. Cervical pain syndromes. In: Maddison PJ, Isenberg DA, Woo P, Glass DN (eds). Oxford Textbook of Rheumatology. Oxford University Press, Oxford, 1993: 1060–1070.
14. Heller CA, Stanley P, Lewis-Jones B, Heller RF. Value of X ray examinations of the cervical spine. Brit Med J 1983; 287: 1276–1278.
15. Johnson MJ, Lucas GL. Value of cervical spine radiographs as a screening tool. Clin Orthop 1997; 340: 102–108.
16. Goodman BW. Neck pain. Primary Care 1988; 15: 689–708.
17. Auten GM, Levy CS, Smoth MA. *Haemophilus parainfluenzae* as a rare cause of epidural abscess. Case report and review. Rev Infect Disc 1991; 13: 609–612.
18. Darouiche RO, Hamill RJ, Greenberg SB, Weathers SW, Muscher DM. Bacterial spinal epidural abscess: review of 43 cases and literature survey. Medicine 1992; 71: 369–385.
19. Danner RL, Hartman RJ. Update of spinal epidural abscess: 35 cases and review of literature. Rev Infect Dis 1987; 9: 265–274.
20. Hlavin ML, Kaminski HJ, Ross JS, Ganz E. Spinal epidural abscess: a ten year perspective. Neurosurgery 1990; 27: 177–184.
21. Verner EF, Musher DM. Spinal epidural abscess. Med Clin North Am 1985; 69: 375–384.
22. Elias M. Cervical epidural abscess following trigger point injection. J Pain Symptom Management 1994; 9: 71–72.
23. Case records of the Massachusetts General Hospital. Case 16-1992. A 27-year-old woman with pain in the neck and shoulder and clumsiness of the hand. New Engl J Med 1992; 326: 1070–1076.
24. Waldman SD. Cervical epidural abscess after cervical epidural nerve block with steroids. Anesth Analg 1991; 72: 717–718.
25. Lasker RB, Harter DH. Cervical epidural abscess. Neurology 1987; 37: 1747–1753.
26. Del Curling O, Gower DJ, McWhorter JM. Changing concepts in spinal epidural abscess: a report of 29 cases. Neurosurgery 1990; 27: 185–192.
27. Vilke GM, Honingford EA. Cervical spine epidural abscess in a patient with no predisposing risk factors. Ann Emerg Med 1996; 27: 777–780.
28. Williams JM, Allegra JR. Spontaneous cervical epidural haematoma. Ann Emerg Med 1994; 23: 1368–1370.
29. Lobitz B, Grate I. Acute epidural hematoma of the cervical spine: an unusual cause of neck pain. South Med J 1995; 88: 580–582.
30. Beatty RM, Winston KR. Spontaneous cervical epidural haematoma: a consideration of etiology. J Neurosurg 1984; 61: 143–148.
31. Matsumae M, Shimoda M, Shibuya N, Veda M, Yamamoto I, Sato O. Spontaneous cervical epidural hematoma. Surg Neurol 1987; 28: 381–384.
32. Hurst PG, Seeger J, Carter P, Marus FI. Value of magnetic resonance imaging for diagnosis of cervical epidural hematoma associated with anticoagulation after cardiac valve replacement. Am J Cardiol 1989; 63: 1016–1017.
33. Mustafa MH, Gallino R. Spontaneous spinal epidural hematoma causing cord compression after streptokinase and heparin therapy for acute coronary artery occlusion. South Med J 1988; 81: 1202–1203.
34. Krolick MA, Cintrom GB. Spinal epidural hematoma causing cord compression after tissue plasminogen activator and heparin therapy. South Med J 1991; 84: 670–671.
35. Rose KD, Croissant PD, Parliament CF, Levin MB. Spontaneous spinal epidural hematoma with associated platelet dysfunction from excessive garlic consumption. Neurosurgery 1990; 26: 880–882.
36. Sharp J, Purser DW, Lawrence JS. Rheumatoid arthritis of the cervical spine in the adult. Ann Rheum Dis 1958; 17: 303–313.

37. Isdale IC, Conlon PW. Atlanto-axial subluxation: a six-year follow-up report. Ann Rheum Disc 1971; 30: 387-389.
38. Hochberg M, Borenstein D, Arnett F. The absence of back pain in classic ankylosing spondylitis. Johns Hopkins Med J 1978; 143: 181-183.
39. Melsom R, Benjamin J, Barnes C. Spontaneous atlanto-axial subluxation: an unusual presenting manifestation of Reiter's syndrome. Ann Rheum Dis 1989; 48: 170-172.
40. Halla JT, Bliznak J, Hardin JG. Involvement of the craniocervical junction in Reiter's syndrome. J Rheumatol 1988; 15: 1722-1725.
41. Bird HA, Esselinckx W, Dixon AStJ, Mowat AG, Wood PHN. An evaluation of criteria for polymyalgia rheumatica. Ann Rheum Dis 1979; 38: 434-439.
42. Fahlgren H. Retropharyngeal tendonitis. Cephalalgia 1986; 6: 169-174.
43. Sarkozi J, Fam AG. Acute calcific retropharyngeal tendonitis: an unusual cause of neck pain. Arthr Rheum 1984; 27: 708-710.
44. Ekbom K, Torhall J, Annell K, Traff J. Magnetic resonance image in retropharyngeal tendonitis. Cephalalgia 1994; 14: 266-269.
45. Karasick D, Karasick S. Calcific retropharyngeal tendonitis. Skeletal Radiol 1981; 7: 203-205.
46. Hartley J. Acute cervical pain associated with retropharyngeal calcium deposit. J Bone Joint Surg 1964; 46A: 1753-1754.
47. Bernstein SA. Acute cervical pain associated with soft-tissue calcium deposition anterior to the interspace of the first and second cervical vertebrae. J Bone Joint Surg 1975; 57A: 426-428.
48. Newmark H, Forrester DM, Brown JC, Robinson A, Olken SM, Bledsoe R. Calcific tendonitis of the neck. Radiology 1978; 128: 355-358.
49. Newmark H, Zee CS, Frankel P, Robinson A, Blau L, Gans DC. Chronic calcific tendonitis of the neck. Skeletal Radiol 1981; 7: 207-208.
50. Fischer RP. Cervical radiographic evaluation of alert patients following blunt trauma. Ann Emerg Med 1984; 13: 905-907.
51. Jacobs LM, Schwartz R. Prospective analysis of acute cervical spine injury: a methodology to predict injury. Ann Emerg Med 1986; 15: 44-49.
52. Mace SE. Emergency evaluation of cervical spine injuries: CT versus plain radiographs. Ann Emerg Med 1985; 14: 973-975.
53. Roberge RJ, Wears RC, Kelly M et al. Selective application of cervical spine radiography in alert victims of blunt trauma: a prospective study. J Trauma 1988; 28: 784-788.
54. McNamara RM. Post-traumatic neck pain: a prospective and follow-up study. Ann Emerg Med 1988; 17: 906-911.
55. Kreipke DL, Gillespie KR, McCarthy MC, Mail JT, Lappas JC, Broadie TA. Reliability of indications for cervical spine films in trauma patients. J Trauma 1989; 29: 1438-1439.
56. Hoffman JR, Schriger DL, Mower W, Luo JS, Zucker M. Low-risk criteria for cervical-spine radiography in blunt trauma: a prospective study. Ann Emerg Med 1992; 21: 1454-1460.
57. Gerrelts BD, Petersen EU, Mabry J, Petersen SR. Delayed diagnosis of cervical spine injuries. J Trauma 1991; 31: 1622-1626.
58. Bachulis BL, Long WB, Hynes GD, Johnson MC. Clinical indications for cervical spine radiographs in the traumatized patient. Am J Surg 1987; 153: 473-477.
59. Mercer S, Bogduk N. Intra-articular inclusions of the cervical synovial joints. Brit J Rheumatol 1993; 32: 705-710.
60. Wortzman G, Dewar FP. Rotatory fixation of the atlantoaxial joint: rotational atlantoaxial subluxation. Radiology 1968; 90: 479-487.
61. Jayakrishnan VK, Teasdale E. Torticollis due to atlanto-axial rotatory fixation following general anaesthesia. Brit J Neurosurg 2000; 14: 583-585.
62. Wise JJ, Cheney R, Fischgrund J. Traumatic bilateral rotatory dislocation of the atlanto-axial joints: a case report and review of the literature. J Spinal Dis 1997; 10: 451-453.
63. Fielding JW, Hawkins RJ. Atlanto-axial rotatory fixation (fixed rotatory subluxation of the atlanto-axial joint). J Bone Joint Surg 1977; 59A: 37-44.
64. Van Holsbeeck EMA, Mackay NNS. Diagnosis of acute atlanto-axial rotatory fixation. J Bone Joint Surg 1989; 71B: 90-91.
65. McKnight P, Friedman J. Torticollis due to cervical epidural abscess and osteomyelitis. Neurology 1992; 42: 696-697.
66. Harinck HI, Buvoet OL, Vellenga CJ, Blanksma HJ, Frijlink WB. Relation between signs and symptoms in Paget's disease of bone. Quart J Med 1986; 58: 133-151.
67. Takano Y, Homma T, Okumura H, Takahashi HE. Ganglion cyst occurring in the ligamentum flavum of the cervical spine: case report. Spine 1992; 17: 1531-1533.
68. Lunardi P, Acqui M, Ricci G, Agrillo A, Ferrante L. Cervical synovial cysts: case report and review of the literature. Eur Spine J 1999; 8: 232-237.
69. Shima Y, Rothman SLG, Yasura K, Takahashi S. Degenerative intraspinal cyst of the cervical spine: case report and literature review. Spine 2002; 27: E18-E22.
70. Gore DR, Sepic SB, Gardner GM. Roentgenographic findings of the cervical spine in asymptomatic people. Spine 1986; 1: 521-524.
71. Elias F. Roentgen findings in the asymptomatic cervical spine. NY State J Med 1958; 58: 3300-3303.
72. Van der Donk J, Schouten JSAG, Passchier J, van Romunde LKJ, Valkenburg HA. The associations of neck pain with radiological abnormalities of the cervical spine and personality traits in a general population. J Rheumatol 1991; 18: 1884-1889.
73. Fridenberg ZB, Miller WT. Degenerative disc disease of the cervical spine: a comparative study of asymptomatic and symptomatic patients. J Bone Joint Surg Am 1963; 45A: 1171-1178.
74. Cherington M, Hendee R. Accessory nerve palsy - a painful cranial neuropathy: surgical cure. Headache 1978; 18: 274-275.
75. Yano K, Murase S, Kuroda T, Noguchi K, Tanabe Y, Yamada H. Cervical cord compression by the vertebral artery causing a severe cervical pain: case report. Surg Neurol 1993; 40: 43-46.
76. Schattner A. Pain in the neck. Lancet 1996; 348: 411-412.
77. Bogduk N, Yoganandan N. Biomechanics of the cervical spine. Part 3: minor injuries. Clin Biomech 2001; 16: 267-275.
78. Wolfe F, Smythe HA, Yunus MB et al. The American College of Rheumatology 1990 criteria for the classification of fibromyalgia: report of the Multicenter Criteria Committee. Arthr Rheum 1990; 33: 160-172.
79. Robinson PJ, Davis JP, Fraser JG. The hyoid syndrome: a pain in the neck. J Laryngol Otol 1994; 108: 855-858.

80. Silbert PL, Makri B, Schievink WI. Headache and neck pain in spontaneous internal carotid and vertebral artery dissections. Neurology 1995; 45: 1517–1522.

81. Biousse V, D'Anglejan-Chatillon J, Massiou H, Bousser MG. Head pain in non-traumatic carotid artery dissection: a series of 65 patients. Cephalalgia 1994; 14: 33–36.

82. Sturzenegger M. Headache and neck pain: the warning symptoms of vertebral artery dissection. Headache 1994; 34: 187–193.

83. Garrard P, Barnes D. Aortic dissection presenting as a neurological emergency. J R Soc Med 1996; 89: 271–272.

84. Hirst AE, Johns VJ, Kime FW. Dissecting aneurysm of the aorta: a review of 505 cases. Medicine 1958; 37: 217–275.

85. Hoffman JR, Schriger DL, Mower W, Luo JS, Zucker M. Low-risk criteria for cervical-spine radiography in blunt trauma: a prospective study. Ann Emerg Med 1992; 21: 1454–1460.

86. Stiell IG, Wells GA, Vandemheen KL et al. The Canadian C-spine rule for radiography in alert and stable trauma patients. JAMA 2001; 286: 1841–1848.

87. Seletz E. Whiplash injuries: neurophysiological basis for pain and methods used for rehabilitation. JAMA 1958; 168: 1750–1755.

88. Signoret F, Feron JM, Bonfait H, Patel A. Fractured odontoid with fractured superior articular process of the axis. J Bone Joint Surg 1986; 68B: 182–184.

89. Craig JB, Hodgson BF. Superior facet fractures of the axis vertebra. Spine 1991; 16: 875–877.

90. Stroobants J, Fidler L, Storms JL, Klaes R, Dua G, van Hoye M. High cervical pain and impairment of skull mobility as the only symptoms of an occipital condyle fracture. J Neurosurg 1994; 81: 137–138.

91. Gershon-Cohen J, Glauser F. Whiplash fractures of cervicodorsal spinous processes. Resemblance to shoveller's fracture. JAMA 1954; 155: 560–561.

92. Bilby L, Santora AH. Prevertebral hematoma secondary to whiplash injury necessitating emergency intubation. Anesth Analg 1990; 70: 112–114.

93. Howcroft AJ, Jenkins DHR. Potentially fatal asphyxia following a minor injury of the cervical spine. J Bone Joint Surg 1977; 59B: 93–94.

94. Spenler CW, Benfield JR. Esophageal disruption from blunt and penetrating external trauma. Arch Surg 1976; 111: 633–637.

95. Hinse P, Thie A, Lachenmayer L. Dissection of the extracranial vertebral artery: report of four cases and review of the literature. J Neurol Neurosurg Psychiat 1991; 54: 863–869.

96. Janjua KJ, Goswami V, Sagar G. Whiplash injury associated with acute bilateral internal carotid arterial dissection. J Trauma 1996; 40: 456–458.

97. Tulyapronchote R, Selhorst JB, Malkoff MD, Gomez CR. Delayed sequelae of vertebral artery dissection and occult cervical fractures. Neurology 1994; 44: 1397–1399.

98. Viktrup L, Knudsen GM, Hansen SH. Delayed onset of fatal basilar thrombotic embolus after whiplash injury. Stroke 1995; 26: 2194–2196.

99. Wosazek GE, Balzer K. Strangulation of the internal carotid artery by the hypoglossal nerve. J Trauma 1990; 30: 332–335.

100. Merskey H, Bogduk N (eds). Classification of Chronic Pain. Descriptions of Chronic Pain Syndromes and Definition of Pain Terms, 2nd edn. IASP Press, Seattle, 1994: 103–111.

101. Australian Acute Musculoskeletal Pain Guidelines Group. Evidence-Based Management of Acute Musculoskeletal Pain. Australian Academic Press, Brisbane, 2003 (Online. Available at http://www.nhmrc.gov.au)

3 Risk factors

KEY POINTS

- The major *etiological risk factors* for neck pain are: educational level, occupation, previous injury, working with machines, and stress at work.

- Psychological factors are conspicuously not major risk factors.

- There are no useful data on the *prognostic risk factors* for neck pain.

For neck pain following whiplash:

- The singular *etiological risk factor* is being involved in a motor vehicle accident that precipitates pain.

- The cardinal *prognostic risk factor* is initial pain intensity.

- Another, but weaker factor is *retaining a lawyer*.

- The available evidence refutes the notion that patients with whiplash exhibit litigation neurosis.

Two types of risk factors apply to neck pain. *Etiological* risk factors are factors evident in asymptomatic individuals that are associated with a statistically greater risk of those individuals developing neck pain. *Prognostic* risk factors are factors exhibited or experienced by patients with acute neck pain that are associated with a statistically greater risk that they will develop chronic neck pain. Both are pertinent to understanding and managing neck pain.

The fact that a risk factor is associated with the incidence of neck pain does not, *per se*, constitute evidence that the factor causes neck pain, for the relationship to neck pain may be indirect. However, if they are a contributing factor to the genesis or maintenance of symptoms, some risk factors may interfere with response to treatment. If they are recognized, and if they are amenable to modification or eradication, reducing or removing these risk factors may improve response to treatment.

ETIOLOGICAL RISK FACTORS

Conspicuous in the literature on risk factors for neck pain is the predominance of *occupational* factors. This might reflect a bias among the investigators, for much of the literature is to be found in occupational medicine journals, but in these studies psychosocial factors have not been ignored. Indeed, some studies have specifically investigated psychosocial factors. In overview, it is apparent that the *factors pertaining to neck pain are different in nature from those pertaining to back pain.* Practitioners should, therefore, not extrapolate to neck pain what they understand to apply to back pain.

An important realization is that while some factors *appear* to be significantly related to neck pain upon univariate analysis, they become insignificant upon multivariate analysis. That means that certain factors seem to be significantly related to neck pain when looked at in isolation, but when the factor is analyzed in the context of other factors the relationship disappears. This occurs when certain risk factors are, in fact, only indirectly related to neck pain, and are themselves a result of more powerful, or overriding factors.

NOT RISK FACTORS

Factors that have been refuted as risk factors for neck pain, for lack of significant correlation or on the grounds of odds ratios barely greater than 1.0 with 95% confidence intervals that range below 1.0, are: degenerative disc disease,[1] zygapophysial osteoarthrosis,[1] smoking,[2] socio-economic status,[3] and prolonged sitting at a work station.[4]

PERSONAL AND OCCUPATIONAL RISK FACTORS

Factors found positively to be associated with neck pain are shown in Table 3.1.

Although working with machines is a risk factor for secretaries, detailed analysis of further possible contributing factors, such as equipment, lumbar support, support of feet, trunk posture, neck posture, hand height, did not reveal any consistent pattern of ergonomic stress that might account for the association between neck pain and working with machines.[5]

Among sewing machine operators there is a clear dose-response relationship in that duration of employment in the industry increases the risk of neck pain.[3,6] For secretaries, there is a trend toward a similar relationship but it is not significant statistically.[4]

In addressing physical risk factors for neck pain, a systematic review[7,8] found that few studies were of high quality. When stringent standards of evidence were applied, the review found that there is some evidence for a positive relationship between neck pain and the duration of sedentary posture at work, and between neck pain and twisting or bending of the trunk at work. If lesser standards of evidence were conceded, some evidence emerged that neck flexion, arm force,

Table 3.1 Risk factors found to be associated with neck pain

Risk factor	Odds ratio	95% confidence interval	Source
Female gender	1.98		1
Educational level			
< 8 years	2.44	1.68–3.55	2
8–12 years	1.7	1.13–2.57	2
Occupation			
professional	1.00		2
clerical	1.78	1.36–2.32	2
industry	2.23	1.70–2.93	2
agriculture	1.97	1.48–2.59	2
Physical stress at work	1.26	1.18–1.33	2
Mental stress at work	1.20	1.12–1.28	2
Previous injury	1.97	1.62–2.38	2
Working with machines	1.65	1.02–2.67	4

arm posture, hand-arm vibration, and workplace design constituted risk factors for neck pain.

A large population study[9] revealed that neck pain of high intensity and associated with disability was strongly associated with co-morbidity, such as low back pain, headaches, cardiovascular disorders, digestive disorders, and a history of motor vehicle collision. However, apart from motor vehicle collision, the relationship applied only to those patients whose health was moderately or severely impaired by back pain, headache, cardiovascular disorders or digestive disorders. This applied to only 26% of the population in the case of back pain, 18% for headache, and less than 10% in the case of cardiovascular and digestive disorders. Thus, the reported relationship applies only to a minority of the population with severe co-morbid disorders.

PSYCHOSOCIAL RISK FACTORS

When they have been investigated, an interesting pattern of psychosocial risk factors for neck pain has emerged. Upon comparing individuals with neck pain with controls, both in manual workers and in office workers, certain specific psychological variables have been found *not* to be significantly different.[10] These include social support, depression, anxiety, coping ability, self-confidence, ability to solve problems, sense of humor, irritability, impatience, psychosis, extroversion or lying, as measured on the Eysenck Personality Questionnaire.

Factors found to be significantly related to neck pain upon univariate analysis in manual workers only include indoor environment, but not activity, neuroticism, workload pace, job control, job instruction, or off-work duties.[10] Conversely among office workers only, significant factors were activity, neuroticism, general tension, psychosomatics, workload pace, workplace design, job control, job instruction, and off-work duties, but not load variation or indoor environment.[10] Upon univariate analysis, general tension was the only variable to be significantly associated with neck pain in both groups of workers.

Upon multivariate analysis, however, the two factors that survived as significant among manual workers were general tension and ability to vary workload. These factors alone correctly classified 87% of the subjects. Among office workers the factors were job control, general tension and psychosomatic symptoms. These factors correctly classified 85% of the subjects.

Although "perceived general tension" was a consistent and significant risk factor for neck pain in the study cited above, this variable was poorly defined. In essence, patients were simply asked to indicate their own perceived level of general tension. It is not clear whether this referred to psychological tension, physical tension, or any combination of both. It is conspicuous, however, that more conventional psychological variables, notably depression and neuroticism, did not emerge as consistent risk factors.

In another study, which ignored occupational factors but compared radiological features and psychological features, factors that emerged as significant risk factors for neck pain were social inadequacy, rigidity and level of injury, but the odds ratios for these factors were less than those for degenerative disc disease and osteoarthrosis as predictors of neck pain.[1] The one psychological factor that emerged as strongly associated with neck pain was inadequacy.[1]

In studies of secretaries, poor psychosocial work environment was found to correlate with neck pain, with an odds ratio of 2.85 with a 95% confidence interval of 1.28 to 6.32.[4,11] The four factors found to constitute a poor psychosocial work environment were lack of co-operation and camaraderie among employees, high workload, lack of possibility to influence one's work, and too great work demands.[11]

A study of sewing machine operators revealed interesting comparative data for risk factors for neck and for other musculoskeletal complaints:[12]

* Economic status, exercise, marital status, children, living conditions, work-load at home and activities outside work were *not related* to any musculoskeletal complaints.
* Previous pain symptoms explained a considerable fraction of the variance for symptoms in the lower extremities but *not for pain in the neck* or shoulders.
* Low back pain was correlated with psychosocial life situation but *neck pain was not.*
* Previous pain symptoms and psychological state were significantly related to neck pain and to shoulder pain upon univariate analysis, *but*
* Upon multivariate analysis, psychological state accounted for only *2% of the variance* in symptoms for neck pain and had no effect on shoulder pain.

Job satisfaction appears to be correlated to neck pain but the relationship is through ergonomic factors such as twisted or bent postures.[13]

However, virtually all studies of risk factors for neck pain have been cross-sectional. The one available prospective study, conducted on 2222 men over 3 years, revealed sobering results.[14] There is *no consistent relationship* between neck pain and psychological factors, as measured by the Middlesex Hospital Questionnaire and the Maudsley Personality Inventory. Such relationships that do emerge do not occur in all occupations. Relationships seen in machine operators are absent in carpenters. Relationships that are seen are weak with odds ratios barely greater than 1.0 whose 95% confidence intervals overlap 1.0. Relationships seen upon univariate analysis disappear upon multivariate analysis.

Psychological factors are not prominent, let alone powerful, predictors of the development of neck pain. Occupational factors dwarf psychological and social factors as predictors of neck pain.

IMPLICATIONS

The available evidence indicates several factors that correlate with neck pain but are not amenable to intervention, such as gender, previous injury, and past education. Probably not amenable to intervention is occupation, in as much as it is unlikely to be possible to convert an industrial or agricultural worker to a professional employee.

Conspicuously absent from the literature on neck pain is evidence of fear-avoidance behavior and bad cognitions, which are operant in back pain. Specific and classical psychological variables have failed to emerge as determinants of neck pain. Such psychological factors as do emerge are vague or intangible, such as general tension and personal inadequacy, which do not lend themselves to formal intervention.

The cardinal determinants of neck pain are work-related, both in a physical domain and in a social domain. Both domains lend themselves to intervention, but both involve rectification of the work environment, not rectification of the patient. In this regard, a laboratory study provided some guidance as to what might be done and what might be effective. Limitation of the daily duration of assembly work was found to be more beneficial than decreasing work pace or increasing breaks from work.[15]

Improving the psychosocial work environment of a patient is not something that can be done through the patient alone. Nor can co-workers and supervisors be instructed to change their behavior as a therapeutic measure for a patient. However, in principle it is possible for a physician, and especially a consultant in occupational medicine, to advise an employer of the risks that their employee's environment confers, and perhaps indicate ways that that environment might be improved for the benefit not only of the patient in question but also for other workers.

REFERENCES

1. Van der Donk J, Schouten JSAG, Passchier J, van Romunde LKJ, Valkenburg HA. The associations of neck pain with radiological abnormalities of the cervical spine and personality traits in a general population. J Rheumatol 1991; 18: 1884-1889.

2. Makela M, Heliovaara M, Sievers K, Impivaara O, Knekt P, Aromaa A. Prevalence, determinants and consequences of chronic neck pain in Finland. Am J Epidemiol 1991; 124: 1356-1367.

3. Andersen JH, Gaardboe O. Prevalence of persistent neck and upper limb pain in a historical cohort of sewing machine operators. Am J Ind Med 1993; 24: 677-687.

4. Kamwendo K, Linton SJ, Moritz U. Neck and shoulder disorders in medical secretaries. Part I. Pain prevalence and risk factors. Scand J Rehab Med 1991; 23: 127-133.

5. Kamwendo K, Linton SJ, Moritz U. Neck and shoulder disorders in medical secretaries. Part II. Ergonomical work environment and symptom profile. Scand J Rehab Med 1991; 23: 135-142.

6. Andersen JH, Gaardboe O. Musculoskeletal disorders of the neck and upper limb among sewing machine operators: a clinical investigation. Am J Ind Med 1993; 24: 689-700.

7. Ariens GAM, Borghouts AJ, Koes BW. Neck pain. In: Crombie IK (ed). Epidemiology of Pain. IASP Press, Seattle, 1999: 235-255.

8. Borghouts JAJ, Koes BW, Bouter LM. The clinical course and prognostic factors of non-specific neck pain: a systematic review. Pain 1998; 77: 1-13.

9. Cote P, Cassidy JD, Carroll L. The factors associated with neck pain and its related disability in the Saskatchewan population. Spine 2000; 25: 1109-1117.

10. Vasseljen O, Westgaard RH, Larsen S. A case-control study of psychological and psychosocial risk factors for shoulder and neck pain at the workplace. Int Arch Occup Environ Health 1995; 66: 375-382.

11. Linton SJ, Kamwendo K. Risk factors in the psychosocial work environment for neck and shoulder pain in secretaries. J Occup Med 1989; 31: 609-613.

12. Westgard RH, Jansen T. Individual and work related factors associated with symptoms of musculoskeletal complaints. II. Different risk factors among sewing machine operators. Brit J Ind Med 1992; 49: 154-162.

13. Tola S, Rihimaaki H, Videman T, Viikari-Juntura E, Hanninen K. Neck and shoulder symptoms among men in machine operating, dynamic physical work and sedentary work. Scand J Work Environ Health 1988; 14: 299-305.

14. Pietri-Taleb F, Riihimaki H, Viikari-Juntura E, Lindstrom K. Longitudinal study on the role of personality characteristics and psychological distress in neck trouble among working men. Pain 1994; 58: 261-267.

15. Mathiassen SE, Winkel J. Physiological comparison of three interventions in light assembly: reduced work pace, increased break allowance and shortened working days. Int Arch Occup Environ Health 1996; 68: 94-108.

PROGNOSTIC RISK FACTORS

A systematic review on this matter,[1,2] found only six studies that reported on prognostic risk factors for neck pain. None, however, provided a statistical analysis that yielded either the relative risk or odds ratio for any association. Consequently, there are no validated prognostic risk factors for neck pain.

REFERENCES

1. Ariens GAM, Borghouts AJ, Koes BW. Neck Pain. In: Crombie IK (ed). Epidemiology of Pain. IASP Press, Seattle, 1999: 235–255.
2. Borghouts JAJ, Koes BW, Bouter LM. The clinical course and prognostic factors of non-specific neck pain: a systematic review. Pain 1998; 77: 1–13.

WHIPLASH

Neck pain following whiplash is complicated by several related factors. When neck pain is subject to compensation, the behavior of patients, and therefore their outcome, may be affected by legislation, administrative regulations and practices, assessment by insurance doctors, lawyers, and the patient's own reactions to these other factors. However, although believed to exist, the influence of these various factors has been difficult to dissect and to demonstrate. And, perhaps ironically, much of the data on neck pain after whiplash suggest that its prognosis is not different from that of uncomplicated neck pain, and indeed may even be better.

ETIOLOGICAL RISK FACTORS

Being involved in a motor vehicle accident is not a risk factor for neck pain. This has been demonstrated in a strong, epidemiological study.[1] That study enrolled 204 subjects who had been in a motor vehicle accident but who did not sustain an injury, and 232 subjects who had been in an accident and developed neck pain attributed to that accident. Each group was matched with a group of subjects (numbering 1599 and 2089, respectively) of similar age and gender who had not been exposed to a motor vehicle accident. All groups were followed for 7 years. The outcome variable was presence of neck pain.

The prevalence of neck pain, at 7 years, in the unexposed groups was 11% and 14.5%, there being no significant difference between these proportions. A similar figure (14%) applied to the exposed group who did not incur an injury. Thus, in subjects exposed to a motor vehicle accident who do not suffer an injury, the prevalence of neck pain in the future is no different from the prevalence in the general community. In contrast, the prevalence in subjects exposed to an accident who did develop symptoms was 39.6%. This difference yields a relative risk of 2.7 (95% CI 2.1–3.5). In essence, being involved in a motor vehicle accident does not increase the risk of developing chronic neck pain, but developing symptoms after a motor vehicle accident increases the risk of chronic neck pain by a factor of three.

PROGNOSTIC RISK FACTORS

A systematic review has carefully addressed the validity of various risk factors that have in the past been considered to be associated with a poor prognosis after whiplash.[2] The singular prognostic factor for adverse outcome is *high initial pain intensity*.[2]

Refuted as prognostic factors were older age, female gender, high acute psychological response, and compensation. There was limited evidence that some other factors *may* be predictive of poorer outcome. These include: sleep disturbance, cognitive impairments, poor concentration, neuroticism, past history of headache, and being unprepared for the collision.[2]

A prospective study, prompted by this review, confirmed but modified the findings of the review.[3] Factors related to poor recovery were female gender, low level of education, high initial neck pain, more severe disability, higher levels of somatization, and sleep difficulties. However, the most consistent predictors of poor recovery were neck pain intensity and work disability.[3]

Other studies have produced additional information. One showed that individual demographic and clinical features did not alone predict poor outcome. However, prognosis was significantly poorer if patients reported a greater number of physical symptoms.[4] Furthermore, how patients cope during the first few weeks after injury is significantly related to the subsequent duration of neck complaints. Thereafter, the intensity of somatic complaints becomes significant.[5]

A systematic series of studies have developed another perspective on prognosis. Case-control studies found that patients with neck pain after whiplash and those with idiopathic neck pain both exhibit mechanical hyperalgesia in the cervical spine and psychological distress.[6,7,8,9] However, what distinguishes patients with chronic neck pain after whiplash is widespread hyperalgesia. These patients exhibit lower thresholds to pressure and to heat pain beyond the neck, in regions such as over the tibialis anterior and over the course of the median nerve and radial nerve.[6,7,8,9] A prospective study showed that predictors of moderate to severe pain and disability at 6 months were high initial neck pain and disability, older age, and hyperalgesia to cold.[10] Predictors of mild pain and disability in the future were high initial pain and disability, psychological distress, and reduced range of movement.[10] Companion studies showed that post-traumatic stress was a feature of patients with chronic neck pain after whiplash, but conspicuously also that fear avoidance behavior was not a feature.[6,7,8]

The emerging picture from these studies is that patients with a poor prognosis are those who initially have higher levels of pain and greater disability, and who do not cope well; but these patients also exhibit hypersensitivity to sensory testing and widespread mechanical hyperalgesia. These latter features are independent of psychological distress,[6,7,8] and implicate central nervous system sensitization in response to persistent pain.

Two recent studies, one retrospective[11] the other prospective,[12] have added another dimension to this picture. In keeping with other studies, they found that the cardinal predictors of poor outcome were low scores on the Bodily Pain and Role Emotional scales of the SF-36 instrument. Those scores reflect greater initial pain that interferes with activity and work, and reduced activity and accomplishments because of emotional problems such as depression or anxiety. The additional feature was that consulting a lawyer was a predictor of poor outcome. That factor persisted as a predictor even when initial pain scores were stratified for severity. That indicates retaining a lawyer has an effect independent of pain severity.

REFERENCES

1. Berglund A, Alfredsson L, Cassidy JD, Jensen I, Nygren A. The association between exposure to a rear-end collision and future neck or shoulder pain: a cohort study. J Clin Epidemiol 2000; 35: 1089–1094.
2. Scholten-Peeters GGM, Verhagen AP, Bekkering GE, van der Windt DAWM, Barnsley L, Oostendorp RAB, Hendriks EJM. Prognostic factors of whiplash-associated disorders: a systematic review of prospective cohort studies. Pain 2003; 104: 303–322.
3. Hendriks EJM, Scholten-Peeters GGM, van der Windt DAWM et al. Prognostic factors for poor recovery in acute whiplash patients. Pain 2005; 114: 408–416.
4. Hartling L, Pickett W, Brison RJ. Derivation of a clinical decision rule for whiplash associated disorders among individuals involved in rear-end collisions. Acc Anal Prev 2002; 34: 531–539.
5. Buitenhuis J, Spanje J, Fidler V. Recovery from acute whiplash: the role of coping styles. Spine 2003; 28: 896–901.
6. Sterling M, Jull G, Vicenzino B, Kenardy J. Sensory hypersensitivity occurs soon after whiplash injury and is associated with poor recovery. Pain 2003; 104: 509–517.
7. Sterling M. A proposed new classification system for whiplash associated disorders: implications for assessment and management. Man Ther 2004; 9: 60–70.
8. Sterling M, Jull G, Vicenzino B, Kenardy J. Characterization of acute whiplash-associated disorders. Spine 2004; 29: 182–188.
9. Scott D, Jull G, Sterling M. Widespread sensory hypersensitivity is a feature of chronic whiplash-associated disorder but not chronic idiopathic neck pain. Clin J Pain 2005; 21: 175–181.
10. Sterling M, Jull G, Vicenzino B, Kennedy J, Darnell R. Physical and psychological factors predict outcome following whiplash injury. Pain 2005; 114: 141–148.
11. Osti OL, Gun RT, Abraham G, Pratt NL, Eckerwall G, Nakamura H. Potential risk factors for prolonged recovery following whiplash injury. Eur Spine J 2005; 14: 90–94.
12. Gun RT, Osti AL, O'Riordan A, Mpelasoka F, Eckerwall CG, Smyth JF. Risk factors for prolonged disability after whiplash injury: a prospective study. Spine 2005; 30: 386–391.

LITIGATION NEUROSIS

"A state of mind, born out of fear, kept alive by avarice, stimulated by lawyers, and cured by a verdict"

Thus did Kennedy[1] define the putative entity called "compensation neurosis." The definition implies that patients complain of persisting symptoms in order to obtain financial gain, in the form of compensation, yet lose their symptoms once compensation has been paid.

Compensation neurosis or litigation neurosis has often been invoked in arguments about whiplash, to explain why patients with neck pain after whiplash fail to recover.[2,3,4,5,6] A survey of physicians in the United States found that over 30% believed that "once litigation is settled, symptoms quickly resolve."[7]

Another epithet that can be applied to this notion is no less engaging linguistically but more closely related to the available evidence:

"A label, born out of ignorance, and kept alive by prejudice."

This notion of compensation neurosis or litigation neurosis did not arise from evidence. It is a convenient label, used to explain chronicity, founded on personal opinion, and sustained by others of the same opinion, despite the absence of evidence.

Even the seminal paper on this topic provides self-defeating data. In his essay on compensation neurosis, Miller[8] described 45 patients with a history of head injury, 41 of whom returned to work after settlement of their claim. Yet these patients were drawn from an inception cohort of 4000 patients, which constitutes a prevalence of only 1%. These data demonstrate that even if compensation neurosis occurs, it is a rare phenomenon.

In contrast to opinions, formal studies and reviews have, by and large, found no evidence of litigation neurosis in patients who suffer whiplash. Competent follow-up studies have found that the prevalence of chronicity is independent of litigation.[9,10,11,12,13] Reviews have found no evidence to support the notion of litigation neurosis.[14,15,16,17]

There is, however, another dimension to this issue. Although there is no evidence that litigation affects the prognosis of patients *within* a given system, there is circumstantial evidence that rates of recovery may differ between systems. A Canadian study found that median times to case closure were significantly shorter under a no-fault system of compensation than under a tort system.[18] The authors concluded that: "the elimination of compensation for pain and suffering is associated with a decreased incidence and improved prognosis of whiplash injury."

The principal problem with this study, however, is that it was based on insurance records rather than on clinically demonstrated recovery. Closure of a claim may be a product of administrative practices, and is not a faithful index of clinical recovery. We cannot be certain, therefore, that a no-fault system actually is associated with a better prognosis.

In effect, therefore, there is basically no evidence to support the notion of litigation neurosis. Although promoted by opinion, it has defied detection when subject to scientific scrutiny.

REFERENCES

1. Kennedy F. The mind of the injured worker: its effect on disability periods. Compens Med 1946; 1: 19–24.
2. Balla JI. The late whiplash syndrome: a study of an illness in Australia and Singapore. Cult Med Psychiat 1982; 6: 191–210.
3. Berry H. Psychological aspects of chronic neck pain following hyperextension-flexion strains of the neck. In: Morley TP (ed). Current Controversies in Neurosurgery. WB Saunders, Philadelphia, 1976: 51–60.
4. Gorman WF. "Whiplash" fictive or factual. Bull Am Acad Psychiatry Law 1979; 7: 245–248.
5. Hodge JR. The whiplash neurosis. Psychosomatics 1971; 12: 245–249.
6. Mills H, Horne G. Whiplash – manmade disease? NZ Med J 1986; 99: 373–374.
7. Evans RW, Evans RI, Sharp MJ. The physician survey on the post-concussion and whiplash syndromes. Headache 1994; 34: 268–274.
8. Miller H. Accident neurosis. BMJ 1961; 1: 919–925, 992–998.
9. Norris SH. Watt I. The prognosis of neck injuries resulting from rear-end vehicle collisions. J Bone Joint Surg 1983; 65B: 608–611.
10. Maimaris C, Barnes MR, Allen MJ. "Whiplash injuries" of the neck: a retrospective study. Injury 1988; 19: 393–396.
11. Pennie B, Agambar L. Patterns of injury and recovery in whiplash. Injury 1991; 22: 57–59.
12. Parmar HV, Raymakers R. Neck injuries from rear impact road traffic accidents: prognosis in persons seeking compensation. Injury 1993; 24: 75–78.
13. Swartzman LC, Teasell RW, Shapiro AP, McDermid AJ. The effect of litigation status on adjustment to whiplash injury. Spine 1996; 21: 53–58.
14. Teasell RW, Shapiro AP. Whiplash injuries: an update. Pain Res Manag 1998; 3: 81–90.
15. Mendelson G. Not "cured by a verdict." Effect of legal settlement on compensation claimants. Med J Aust 1982; 2: 132–134.
16. Mendelson G. Follow-up studies of personal injury litigants. Int J Law Psychiat 1984; 7: 179–188.
17. Shapiro AP, Roth RS. The effect of litigation on recovery from whiplash. In: Teasell R, Shapiro A (eds). Spine: State of the Art Reviews. Cervical Flexion-Extension/Whiplash Injuries. Hanley and Belfus, Philadelphia, 1993, 7: 551–556.
18. Cassidy JD, Carrol LJ, Cote P, Lemstra M, Berglund A, Nygren A. Effect of eliminating compensation for pain and suffering on the outcome of insurance claims for whiplash injury. New Engl J Med 2000; 342: 1179–1186.

PART

2 Acute neck pain

Acute neck pain: natural history

KEY POINTS

Good prospective data on the natural history of neck pain are lacking, but:

- the prognosis of acute neck pain is largely favorable

- some 40% of patients can expect to recover fully

- a further 25% will retain only mild symptoms.

Of patients with acute neck pain following whiplash:

- some 80% can expect to recover rapidly, and be fully recovered within a year.

In principle, knowing the natural history of neck pain is pertinent for two reasons. For academic purposes, it establishes a baseline against which the apparent effectiveness of any treatment can be assessed; if the natural history of the complaint is favorable, it will account for much of the apparent effectiveness of treatment. For practical purposes, if the natural history is favorable, practitioners can reassure their patients that they will recover in time. Reassurance, therefore, is not a gratuitous exercise, but becomes an active intervention based on sound epidemiological evidence.

It transpires, however, there are very few data on the natural progression of either acute or chronic neck pain that is left untreated. Authorities that have wrestled with this issue have largely resorted to surrogate data, relying on studies of treatment to infer that the outcomes in the control group reflect the natural history of the condition.[1,2]

SURROGATE DATA

Two problems arise with the use of surrogate data from clinical trials. Firstly, they do not exclude non-specific treatment effects. Treatment, even with placebo or sham therapy, constitutes an intervention that may hasten natural recovery.

Secondly, such data, in the case of neck pain, stem from studies of small samples, which may not reflect the general population.

Even allowing for these factors, the surrogate data on neck pain paint an indistinct or incomplete picture.[1,2] Few studies have explicitly studied either acute neck pain or chronic neck pain; most enrolled mixed populations. Most had limited periods of follow-up, with median times of less than 3 months. Although patients improve, the proportion that does so ranges from 10% to 100%, with an average of 30–50%, depending on the study.

OBSERVATIONAL STUDIES

In a retrospective study, Gore et al.[3] reviewed the status of 205 patients seen at least 10 years previously for complaints of neck pain without neurologic deficits and not due to malignancy or rheumatoid arthritis. Patients were asked to describe their pain as:

- mild if it was present but easily tolerated and did not interfere with performance of activities of daily living
- moderate if it was tolerable but interfered with some activities of daily living
- severe if it was not well tolerated and significantly interfered with activities.

The evolution of complaints is summarized in Table 4.1. The data do not indicate what happened to individual patients, or how patients in particular initial categories progressed, but they do indicate that neck pain is relatively benign in as much as 43% of patients recover fully within 10 years. On the other hand, neck pain is not totally benign, since some 25% of patients continue to have moderate symptoms and some 7% remain or become severely disabled.

Table 4.1 Evolution of neck pain in 205 patients over 10 years. Based on Gore et al.[3]

	Initial status		Status after 10 years	
Pain rating	Number	%	Number	%
None	0	0	89	43
Mild	27	13	51	25
Moderate	81	40	51	25
Severe	97	47	14	7
Total	205	100	205	100

These data, however, are somewhat confounded in that 121 of the 205 patients suffered neck pain after injury, 76 as a result of a motor vehicle accident, and the remainder as a result of some other form of accident. Consequently, the picture that they depict may not be generalizable, if the natural history of patients with post-traumatic neck pain differs from that of patients with idiopathic neck pain.

The limited data that are available suggest that this may not be the case. A British study[4] reviewed, in 1961 or 1962, 51 patients with neck pain who attended a neurology department in 1947, who had no neurological signs, and who were accorded a diagnosis of cervical spondylosis on the basis of cervical radiographic investigation. When reviewed between 2 and 19 years after onset of symptoms, 22 (44%) patients had no symptoms, 15 had only mild or intermittent symptoms, and 14 (28%) had troublesome symptoms or moderate disability. There was no apparent difference in effect of treatment by collar, exercises, manipulation, rest or no therapy. Like that of Gore et al.,[3] this study indicates that some 40% of patients with neck pain recover fully in due course, and a further 25% or so remain with only mild symptoms.

WHIPLASH

Whiplash attracts an unsavory reputation. Some pundits believe that because neck pain after whiplash is potentially compensable, patients maintain their symptoms and do not recover. The epidemiological literature, however, refutes this. Indeed, it shows that the natural history of acute neck pain following whiplash is generally favorable and, if anything, is better than that of acute neck pain not due to whiplash.

Some studies that have attempted to record the natural history of acute neck pain after whiplash[5,6,7,8] have suffered from small inception cohorts and dwindling numbers, with the result that the confidence intervals of the proportions of patients showing recovery or persistence of pain are quite large.[9] This prevents meaningful figures being derived from the study.[9]

Studies that have used claims data from insurance companies would suggest that the natural progression of acute neck pain after whiplash is very favorable, with the vast majority (97%)[10] having recovered by 12 months. However, such recovery rates are based on claims closure and certified "work-readiness," not on clinically demonstrated recovery.

Actual clinical data were obtained in a Swiss study that recruited patients with acute neck pain after whiplash, from family care practitioners, as soon as possible after injury.[11] These patients showed rapid recovery with the passage of time (Figure 4.1). Some 56% had fully

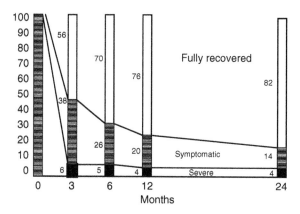

Figure 4.1 The percentage of patients with acute neck pain after whiplash achieving different grades of recovery with the passage of time. Based on Radanov et al.[11]

recovered by 3 months, 70% by 6 months, 76% by 1 year, and 82% by 2 years. At these same points in time, the proportion of patients still having mild or moderate symptoms fell from 38%, to 26%, 20% and 14%. Some 5% of patients remained in severe pain throughout the period of follow-up.

These data indicate that acute neck pain after whiplash is essentially a benign disorder from which most patients can expect to recover fully. This has been reinforced by a clinical study in which the intervention group were offered a short course of analgesics but then encouraged to resume normal activities with no further formal treatment.[12] At 6 months and 1 year, only 15% of patients continued to have chronic neck pain.

IMPLICATIONS

In the light of these data, practitioners can be confident when reassuring patients. The data show that the natural history of acute neck pain, particularly after whiplash, is favorable and that most patients can expect to recover simply with the passage of time. Practitioners can share this information with their patients, and can be honest when reassuring them. That reassurance constitutes evidence-based practice.

References

1. Ariens GAM, Borghouts AJ, Koes BW. Neck pain. In: Crombie IK (ed). Epidemiology of Pain. IASP Press, Seattle, 1999: 235–255.
2. Borghouts JAJ, Koes BW, Bouter LM. The clinical course and prognostic factors of non-specific neck pain: a systematic review. Pain 1998; 77: 1–13.
3. Gore DR, Sepic SB, Gardner GM, Murray MP. Neck pain: a long-term follow-up of 205 patients. Spine 1987; 12: 1–5.
4. Lees F, Turner JWA. Natural history and prognosis of cervical spondylosis. Brit Med J 1963; 2: 1607–1610.
5. Gargan MF, Bannister GC. Long-term prognosis of soft-tissue injuries of the neck. J Bone Joint Surg 1990; 72B: 901–903.
6. Gargan MF, Bannister GC. The rate of recovery following whiplash injury. Eur Spine J 1994; 3: 162–164.
7. Squires B, Gargan MF, Bannister GC. Soft tissue injuries of the cervical spine: 15-year follow-up. J Bone Joint Surg 1996; 78B: 955–957.
8. Norris SH, Watt I. The prognosis of neck injuries resulting from rear-end vehicle collisions. J Bone Joint Surg 1983; 65B: 608–611.
9. Barnsley L, Lord S, Bogduk N. The pathophysiology of whiplash. In: Malanga GA (ed). Cervical Flexion-Extension/Whiplash Injuries. Spine: State of the Art Reviews. Hanley and Belfus, Philadelphia, 1998; 12: 209–242.
10. Spitzer WO, Skovron ML, Salmi LR et al. Scientific monograph of the Quebec Task Force on Whiplash-Associated Disorders: redefining "whiplash" and its management. Spine 1995; 20 (Suppl 8): 1S–73S.
11. Radanov BP, Sturzenegger M, Di Stefano G. Long-term outcome after whiplash injury: a 2-year follow-up considering features of injury mechanism and somatic, radiologic, and psychosocial findings. Medicine 1995; 74: 281–297.
12. Borchgrevink GE, Kaasa A, McDonagh D, Stiles TC, Haraldseth O, Lereim I. Acute treatment of whiplash neck sprain injuries: a randomized trial of treatment during the first 14 days after a car accident. Spine 1998; 23: 25–31.

Acute neck pain: taking a history

KEY POINTS

- A patho-anatomic diagnosis of neck pain is unlikely to be made on the basis of history alone.

- However, taking a thorough history serves to exclude or to reveal the possibility of a serious cause of neck pain.

- A thorough history can be prompted by a checklist.

- Recording null responses to a checklist serves to protect the practitioner, showing that no potentially significant matters have been overlooked.

Taking a history is the *single most important action* in assessing a patient with acute neck pain. It is from the history that clues pointing to potentially important diagnoses can be obtained. However, no system or protocol for taking a history has been subjected to scientific scrutiny in order to determine either its reliability or its validity. Consequently, taking a history remains more a craft than a science, and is based on tradition and wisdom gained from experience.

One system that has been described is one that has served well for the assessment of headache.[1] Both systematic and comprehensive, it invites an enquiry into several variables that pertain to headache (Box 5.1), but which, in principle and with some adaptations, potentially apply to any form of pain, neck pain being no exception.

CATEGORIES OF ENQUIRY

Site of pain

It is important to establish that the patient does, indeed, complain of neck pain: that what the patient indicates is consistent with the definition of cervical spinal pain (see Chapter 1). Competing alternatives include pain in the throat, suggestive of visceral disease rather than a cervical problem, and headache. Whereas upper cervical pain can be referred to the head, the reverse is also true. Patients with headache can have pain spreading into the neck. The distinction may be difficult, but it can be important, particularly for recognizing vascular conditions that may cause headache, neck pain, or both.

If the patient identifies a reasonably circumscribed area of pain, its location can be used to formulate a prima facie judgment of its segmental origin. If the pain is located in the upper half of the neck, its origin is most likely from the upper cervical segments, with C2–3 being the most likely segment.[4–10] If the pain is located in the lower half of the neck, its origin is probably from the lower cervical segments, with C5–6 and C6–7 being the most likely.[4–10]

Radiation

Neck pain can be referred to the head, upper limb girdle, or chest wall. Referral is a normal feature of spinal pain, and in itself is not diagnostic. However, if a patient has a circumscribed area of pain that they can define well, it may correspond to one of the areas of referred pain known to occur in normal volunteers (Chapter 1). In that event, the pattern of referral can be used to judge, not the source of pain, but at least its approximate segmental location.

In interpreting maps of referred pain, what is not critical is the total distribution or the extent of its boundaries. Critical is where the patient feels the core of their pain; where they feel it most consistently, even though it radiates; and where they feel it worst.[2,3] These features define the epicentre or centroid of

the pain, and it is this that should be correlated with pain maps in order to estimate the spinal segments involved (Figure 5.1).

Patients with pain arising from C2–3 tend to feel that their pain starts in the suboccipital area. That pain may radiate further, into the occiput or to the forehead, but the centre from which it radiates is in the suboccipital area. Similarly, irrespective of where or how far it radiates, pain arising from C3–4 tends to start over the posterolateral neck, more or less over the course of the levator scapulae. Pain from C4–5 characteristically seems to start, or be maximal, over the angle between the neck and the top of the shoulder girdle. Pain from C5–6 concentrates over the supraspinous fossa, before spreading into the deltoid region. Pain from C6–7 can resemble that from C5–6 but will tend to gravitate to the medial border of the scapula.

It must be realized that these patterns do not identify the anatomical source or the cause of pain. They reflect only the neurology of that pain. The patterns are determined by the nerves that supply the source, not by the source itself. Thus, all structures innervated by C5,6—be they zygapophysial joints, discs, or muscles—will present with a similar segmental pattern of referral.

Referred pain *from* the neck, however, must be distinguished from referred pain *to* the neck. Neck pain can be referred to the anterior chest, but the opposite can also occur. Neck pain referred to the chest can

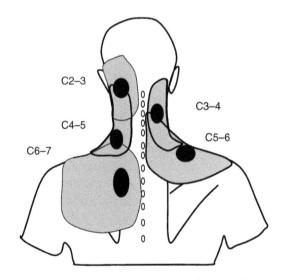

Figure 5.1 Centroids for the segmental origin of referred pain from the cervical spine. The shaded areas indicate the typical zones of referral, from the segments indicated, in normal volunteers and patients. The dark areas represent the centroids, or core areas, where patients feel the pain maximally when it arises from the segment indicated.

mimic angina, and has been called cervical angina.[11,12] Pain arising from the heart or the thoracic aorta may be referred to the neck, but archetypically the chest pain should be worse than the neck pain, and more importantly, the chest pain should be accompanied by associated features indicative of a cardiovascular disorder, such as physical distress, cyanosis, abnormal blood pressure and heart rate, or a bruit.

Somatic referred pain from the cervical spine needs to be distinguished from *radicular pain*, for the subsequent investigation and treatment of the two conditions differ substantially. Unfortunately, the distinction between these two conditions has not been comprehensively studied. Instead, it has been assumed either that practitioners intuitively know the difference between the two, or that all pain radiating into the upper limb is radicular pain. Neither assumption is correct.

From what is known about the nature of somatic referred pain, both from studies in normal volunteers[2,13,14] and from studies of patients,[4,6–10] certain general guidelines can be formulated. Somatic referred pain is perceived as a deep, aching pain, sometimes like an expanding pressure that spreads into the upper limb. Most often, if not typically, it radiates only into the shoulder girdle or proximal arm. Referral into the forearm and hand is possible in principle, and such distal referral has been shown in normal volunteers;[13,14] but it has yet to be shown in patients. Most conspicuously, somatic referred pain is *not associated* with neurological signs.

Radicular pain shares with somatic referred pain the feature that it is perceived in the shoulder girdle and proximal upper limb. It differs, however, in that more often it extends distally into the forearm and hand, especially when the C6 and C7 nerves are affected.[15,16] Most characteristically, although not necessarily always, radicular pain is accompanied by the features of radiculopathy (i.e. paresthesiae, numbness, weakness, and loss of reflexes), each in a dermatomal or myotomal distribution.[16]

Accordingly, if the pain is referred distally into the upper limb, it is likely to be radicular in origin, especially if accompanied by neurological signs. Pain restricted to the shoulder girdle or proximal upper limb is more likely, in the first instance, to be somatic referred pain, especially if there are no neurological signs.

Duration of illness

Establishing how long the neck pain has been present serves two purposes. First, it identifies patients with a sudden, recent onset of pain. This sets the scene for further enquiry under subsequent categories (see below). Second, it determines if the patient has acute or chronic pain (Chapter 1). With respect to management, the evidence-base for acute neck pain is distinctly different from that for chronic neck pain. Establishing which of the two the patient has predicates what interventions are appropriate.

Circumstances of onset

This category of enquiry complements mode of onset (see below) but is different from that category. The circumstances of onset pertain to what else was happening when the neck pain started, or what transpired shortly before that. The obvious relevant circumstances concern trauma.

A history of injury is both alerting and reassuring. It is alerting because fractures become a possible cause of the pain. It is reassuring in that, given an injury, the patient has an attributable cause of their pain, even if it might be difficult to identify.

No history of trauma may be reassuring in that the risk of fracture is low, but it is also disconcerting. If one assumes that it is not natural for a patient to develop neck pain for no reason, the spontaneous onset of pain raises the need to be vigilant for a sinister, red flag condition (Chapter 2).

If there is a history of trauma, its nature should be determined. Attention should be paid to whether the injury was external or inertial—i.e. whether the head or neck were struck, or struck something, or whether the neck sustained an impulse from the trunk without the head or neck striking anything—together with some sense of the magnitude of the forces involved. Fractures of the cervical spine become more likely with external injuries, and less likely with inertial injuries. In both circumstances, fractures are more likely the greater the magnitude of forces involved (see Chapter 7).

A history of viral illness during the preceding week or so may be a risk factor for retropharyngeal tendonitis. Some patients who have had this condition diagnosed reported that they have indeed recently suffered a "flu-like" illness. Unfortunately so few cases of this condition have been studied that the validity of this clue is unknown.

Under this category it is convenient to explore risk factors for spinal infection. These include recent surgery, instrumentation, body penetration (including medical and illicit injections), or concomitant infection elsewhere. Although no data are available as to the validity of these factors in the diagnosis of cervical spinal infection, they are proffered as wisdom-based, and on the basis of retrospective analysis of the histories of patients who were found to have spinal infection. In such cases, it is often conspicuous that a history of body penetration, or recent illness, were available early in the course of events but were not identified at that time. Only later, in retrospect, did it become evident that there were, indeed, grounds for suspecting an infection.

An important consideration is risk factors for aneurysms. Aneurysms may be spontaneous, but they can also be precipitated by periods of prolonged rotation and extension of the neck. A recent history of spinal manipulation is a paramount clue for considering traumatic aneurysm as the source of neck pain.

Mode of onset

This category seeks to establish exactly how the pain came on. The distinction lies in the rate of onset. Most alarming and alerting is the sudden onset of severe pain. Traditional wisdom maintains that this mode of onset is highly sensitive for serious conditions such as fractures and aneurysms; but it is not specific, for those conditions can also have a prolonged or smoldering mode of onset. Explicit quantitative data to this effect are, however, lacking.

A gradual onset over less than a few days, together with a rapid worsening of pain, is a probable sign of acute inflammation. It is characteristic of the onset of retropharyngeal tendonitis, which is a proven, albeit rare, inflammatory condition. Other inflammatory conditions of the cervical spine, however, have not been studied and described with respect to mode of onset. Osteomyelitis, in contrast, has a slow and quiet onset of pain, to the extent that 3 months is not atypical of the time taken to consider and make this diagnosis.

Quality

Most patients with neck pain will describe their pain, if they can, as dull, aching, or pressure-like. This is characteristic of somatic pain. Such a description is not diagnostic of any particular source or cause. Effectively, it is the default description of neck pain.

In contrast, shooting or lancinating pain is not a feature of somatic pain of musculoskeletal origin. Rather, it is strongly suggestive of a neurogenic origin. Neck pain is rarely neurogenic in origin (see Chapter 2), but in those case reports in which a neurogenic cause has been verified, the patient's history included a descriptor such as "shooting" pain.[17]

Severity

Severity is a capricious dimension of pain. One cannot validly distinguish severe pain due to serious pathology from pain that is reportedly severe because the patient is distressed. Severe pain that is sudden in onset is regarded as a warning feature of serious pathology, such as aneurysm; but its sensitivity and specificity as an indicator of serious pathology has not been established.

Otherwise, there is merit in recording the severity of pain, using a visual analogue scale or a numerical pain-rating scale, in order to obtain baseline data. That information becomes valuable later, when assessing the progress of patients. If interventions or the passage of time are successful, there should be a fall in the numerical value assigned to the severity of pain. Comparing follow-up values with baseline values allows the reduction in pain to be quantified.

Frequency

Frequency or periodicity is one of the least relevant categories of enquiry for neck pain. Somatic pain is constant in nature. If intermittent, it does not exhibit any particular, constant periodicity. Intermittent somatic pain is more likely related to precipitating factors or aggravating factors.

Paroxysmal pain, however, is almost diagnostic of neurogenic pain. Although neck pain is rarely neurogenic in origin, when it has been, its paroxysmal nature has been a feature in the history.[17]

Duration

Duration pertains to how long the pain lasts once it starts. Like frequency, duration is of little relevance in the diagnosis of somatic neck pain. Patients will vary as to whether their pain is constant, or lasts only for set periods. No valid inferences can be drawn from this variable. Brief bursts of pain are similarly not diagnostic of a cause, but if part of a paroxysm of pain, they are highly suggestive of a neurogenic origin.

Time of onset

Although time of onset can be relevant in the clinical diagnosis of other forms of pain, it is virtually irrelevant in the context of neck pain. However, its reciprocal can be of relevance—when it fails to abate. Of particular significance is pain that occurs or persists during sleep. Traditional wisdom maintains that this can be a sign of a sinister disorder. In a qualitative sense, that may be a worthwhile guideline, but quantitative data as to the sensitivity or specificity of this feature are lacking.

Precipitating factors

Establishing what brings the pain on serves little purpose with respect to making a diagnosis of neck pain. Most patients will typically describe various movements that can bring on the pain. Some might even venture to demonstrate the effect, without being prompted to do so.

More alerting, however, is when a patient knows what will bring on their pain, or will severely aggravate it, and consciously and deliberately avoids those movements.

Such patients risk being interpreted cynically as hysterical or exaggerating. However, apprehension and caution can be responses to serious instability. Anxiously avoiding rotation of the head can be a feature of atlanto-axial instability, as occurs with odontoid fractures or tears of the alar ligaments.[18]

Aggravating factors

Like precipitating factors, factors that aggravate the pain are of little diagnostic value in the assessment of neck pain. Patients will describe a variety of combinations of movements that can aggravate their pain. No movement pattern has been shown to be diagnostic of any particular source or cause of neck pain.

More disconcerting is the patient who lacks aggravating factors. This suggests a deep-seated cause of pain, such as a vascular lesion or a lesion within a vertebral body, which is not irritated mechanically by movement. However, the validity of this inference is not known.

Relieving factors

Some practitioners might choose to draw inferences about the source or cause of neck pain based on whether it is relieved by certain maneuvers or positions, such as lying down. Such inferences are not valid, and basically amount to no more than finding that the patient has so-called "mechanical" neck pain.

Disconcerting is pain that is not relieved by any measure. Genuinely intractable pain can be a sign of a serious, if not progressive, disorder, particularly if the pain is of recent onset. But intractable pain needs to be distinguished from pain that the patient describes in exaggerated terms in order to emphasize their distress.

An untested, and unpublished, proposition is that patients with a really serious cause of pain tend to look ill, and are withdrawn rather than extrovert about their pain; they are silent rather than vocal in their suffering, as if they "know" in themselves that something is seriously wrong, and do not feel the need to tell everyone.

ASSOCIATED FEATURES

It is with respect to associated features that the most critical, discriminating features of different causes of neck pain can be found. The pursuit of associated features explores what else, apart from the pain, is going wrong. A systematic approach can be taken by incorporating the enquiry into a systems review.

In the following guidelines, where evidence for particular features is available in the context of neck pain, it is cited. Otherwise, the guidelines are based on traditional medical wisdom and teaching, or on similar principles established for back pain.

Past history of illness

A past history of cancer constitutes prima facie grounds for considering metastatic disease.

Immunosuppression, diabetes mellitus, cirrhosis, AIDS, steroid use, recent or concurrent infection are considered risk factors for spinal infection, as are recent body penetration such as catheterization, injections, surgical procedures, and illicit drug use.[19]

General health

Unexplained weight loss is a cardinal cue to consider neoplastic disease.

Fever or night sweats demand consideration of infection or neoplastic disease. Fever, however, is a feature of spinal osteomyelitis in only about 43% of cases.[20]

Exposure

Although the possibilities are rare and remote, it takes little effort to enquire about unusual circumstances that can be associated with exposure to exotic or unusual organisms in the course of occupational or recreational pursuits. A prime example is exposure to hydatid in rural areas. Another is overseas travel to environments that pose a risk for unusual infections.

Nervous system

Numbness or weakness in the extremities suggests radiculopathy, myelopathy, or a central nervous system lesion, and immediately converts the presentation from one of neck pain to one of a neurological disorder.

Headache and vomiting are alerting features of an intracranial lesion.[21]

Disturbances in vision, speech, or balance, in the form of transient ischemic attacks, are cardinal features of aneurysms of the vertebral or internal carotid artery.[22,23,24] Although perhaps not present initially, these features will usually manifest soon after the onset of neck pain. Therefore, it is their subsequent onset to which practitioners should be alerted.

Cardiovascular system

Risk factors for cardiovascular disease raise the probability of an aneurysm being the cause of neck pain.

Use of anticoagulants is a risk factor for cerebral or spinal hemorrhage.[21,25,26,27,28]

Urinary system

Frequency or dysuria may suggest a concomitant urinary tract infection as a source of spinal infection.

Impaired stream raises the possibility of prostatic cancer and spinal metastases.

Endocrine system

Use of steroids is a risk factor not only for spinal infection but also for osteoporosis and pathological fracture.

Although there may be no other clinical cues, hyperparathyroidism can cause osteitis fibrosa, which can be an occult cause of bone pain.

Gastrointestinal system

Unexplained loss of weight gives serious cause to consider a neoplastic cause of neck pain.

Dysphagia can be a sign of a prevertebral cervical lesion.

Musculoskeletal system

Pain in other regions is a cue to consider systemic arthropathy or a systemic inflammatory disorder.

Skin

Skin infections are a risk factor for spinal infection.

Rashes may be indicative of a spondylarthropathy.

Reproductive system

Disorders of the breast or uterus, past or present, invite consideration of neoplastic disease.

Respiratory system

Although respiratory disorders are common and may be incidental, it would be remiss not to consider the possibility of metastatic lung cancer in a patient with chronic cough.

CHECKLIST

For the purposes of ensuring that all potentially relevant matters have been addressed in the history, a checklist can be used (Figure 5.2). This checklist prompts enquiry, and serves to record conveniently not only the responses but also that all matters have been checked. The latter serves to some degree to protect practitioners against possible accusations that they did not bother to enquire fully about a patient's complaint.

In the event that a patient offers a positive response to any matter, that response and the complaint should be pursued along conventional medical lines, and recorded separately. The default expectation, however, is that most patients with neck pain will offer a null response to all items. Such a response serves to indicate and to record that the patient is very unlikely to have a serious condition that is responsible for their neck pain.

Unfortunately, this checklist has only face validity. For acute low back pain in primary care, some data are available as to the sensitivity and specificity of certain features of history as indicators of cancer and infection.[29] Such data have not been collected and reported explicitly for neck pain. It is for this reason that taking a history of neck pain is not based on any scientific evidence. It is based only on traditional wisdom and recommendations drawn from occasional case reports.

The major liability, however, lies not in the lack of science. It lies in practitioners neglecting to take a thorough history, and ignoring such wisdom as is available.

Name: _____				Neck pain			
D.O.B. _____				M.R.N. _____			
Trauma	Y	N	**Neurological**		Endocrine		
Fever	Y	N	Symptoms/signs	Y	N	Corticosteroids	Y	N
Night sweats	Y	N	Cerebrovascular	Y	N	Diabetes	Y	N
Recent surgery	Y	N	Vomiting	Y	N	Hyperparathyroid	Y	N
Catheterization	Y	N	**Cardiovascular**		**GIT**		
Venipuncture	Y	N	Risk factors	Y	N	Dysphagia	Y	N
Illicit drug use	Y	N	Anticoagulants	Y	N	**Musculoskeletal**		
Immunosuppression	Y	N	**Urinary**		Pain elsewhere	Y	N
Awkward posture	Y	N	UTI	Y	N	**Skin**		
Manipulation	Y	N	Hematuria	Y	N	Infections	Y	N
History of cancer	Y	N	Retention	Y	N	Rashes	Y	N
Weight loss	Y	N	**Reproductive**		**Respiratory**		
Exotic exposure	Y	N	Uterine	Y	N	Cough	Y	N
(Overseas) travel	Y	N	Breast	Y	N	**Signature:**		
Comments							
					Date:		

Figure 5.2 A checklist for red flag clinical indicators for neck pain, suitable for inclusion in medical records.

References

1. Lance JW. Mechanism and Management of Headache, 5th edn. Butterworth Heinemann, Oxford, 1993: 31–38.
2. Dwyer A, Aprill C, Bogduk N. Cervical zygapophysial joint pain patterns I: a study in normal volunteers. Spine 1990; 15: 453–457.
3. Aprill C, Dwyer A, Bogduk N. Cervical zygapophyseal joint pain patterns II: a clinical evaluation. Spine 1990; 15: 458–461.
4. Fukui S, Ohseto K, Shiotani M et al. Referred pain distribution of the cervical zygapophyseal joints and cervical dorsal rami. Pain 1996; 68: 79–83.
5. Lord SM, Bogduk N. The cervical synovial joints as sources of post-traumatic headache. J Musculoskelet Pain 1996; 4: 81–94.
6. Schellhas KP, Smith MD, Gundry CR, Pollei SR. Cervical discogenic pain: prospective correlation of magnetic resonance imaging and discography in asymptomatic subjects and pain sufferers. Spine 1996; 21: 300–312.
7. Grubb JA, Kelly CK. Cervical discography: clinical implications from twelve years' experience. Spine 2000; 25: 1382–1389.
8. Bogduk N, Marsland A. The cervical zygapophysial joints as a source of neck pain. Spine 1988; 13: 610–617.
9. Barnsley L, Lord SM, Wallis BJ, Bogduk N. The prevalence of chronic cervical zygapophysial joint pain after whiplash. Spine 1995; 20: 20–26.
10. Lord S, Barnsley L, Wallis BJ, Bogduk N. Chronic cervical zygapophysial joint pain after whiplash: a placebo-controlled prevalence study. Spine 1996; 21: 1737–1745.
11. Booth RE, Rothman RH. Cervical angina. Spine 1976; 1: 28–32.
12. Brodsky AE. Cervical angina: a correlative study with emphasis on the use of coronary arteriography. Spine 1985; 10: 699–709.
13. Kellgren JH. On the distribution of pain arising from deep somatic structures with charts of segmental pain areas. Clin Sci 1939; 4: 35–46.
14. Feinstein B, Langton JBK, Jameson RM, Schiller F. Experiments on referred pain from deep somatic tissues. J Bone Joint Surg 1954; 36A: 981–997.
15. Slipman CW, Plastaras CT, Palmitier RA, Huston CW, Sterenfeld EB. Symptom provocation of fluoroscopically guided cervical nerve root stimulation: are dynatomal maps identical to dermatomal maps? Spine 1998; 23: 2235–2242.
16. Bogduk N. Medical Management of Acute Cervical Radicular Pain. An Evidence-Based Approach. Newcastle Bone and Joint Institute, Newcastle, 1999; 5–11.
17. Yano K, Murase S, Kuroda T, Noguchi K, Tanabe Y, Yamada H. Cervical cord compression by the vertebral artery causing a severe cervical pain: case report. Surg Neurol 1993; 40: 43–46.
18. Dvorak J, Hayek J, Zehnder R. CT-functional diagnostics of the rotatory instability of the upper cervical spine. Part 2. An evaluation on healthy adults and patients with suspected instability. Spine 1987; 12: 726–731.
19. Vilke GM, Honingford FA. Cervical spine epidural abscess in a patient with no predisposing risk factors. Ann Emerg Med 1996; 27: 777–780.
20. Goodman BW. Neck pain. Primary Care 1988; 15: 689–708.
21. Schattner A. Pain in the neck. Lancet 1996; 348: 411–412.
22. Silbert PL, Makri B, Schievink WI. Headache and neck pain in spontaneous internal carotid and vertebral artery dissections. Neurology 1995; 45: 1517–1522.
23. Biousse V, D'Anglejan-Chatillon J, Massiou H, Bousser MG. Head pain in non-traumatic carotid artery dissection: a series of 65 patients. Cephalalgia 1994; 14: 33–36.
24. Sturzenegger M. Headache and neck pain: the warning symptoms of vertebral artery dissection. Headache 1994; 34: 187–193.
25. Hurst PG, Seeger J, Carter P, Marus FI. Value of magnetic resonance imaging for diagnosis of cervical epidural hematoma associated with anticoagulation after cardiac valve replacement. Am J Cardiol 1989; 63: 1016–1017.
26. Mustafa MH, Gallino R. Spontaneous spinal epidural hematoma causing cord compression after streptokinase and heparin therapy for acute coronary artery occlusion. South Med J 1988; 81: 1202–1203.
27. Krolick MA, Cintrom GB. Spinal epidural hematoma causing cord compression after tissue plasminogen activator and heparin therapy. South Med J 1991; 84: 670–671.
28. Rose KD, Croissant PD, Parliament CF, Levin MB. Spontaneous spinal epidural hematoma with associated platelet dysfunction from excessive garlic consumption. Neurosurgery 1990; 26: 880–882.
29. Bogduk N, McGuirk B. Evidence-Based Management of Acute and Chronic Low Back Pain. Elsevier, London, 2002; 33–36.

Acute neck pain: physical examination

KEY POINTS

- Although commonly practiced, physical examination of the neck has no diagnostic value for the identification of musculoskeletal disorders of the cervical spine.

- The reliability of tenderness over the zygapophysial joints is good but lacks any validity.

- The reliability of muscle tenderness varies according to both the observer and the muscle or region tested, and lacks validity.

- Testing of gross ranges of motion has not been tested for reliability, and lacks any validity.

- Provocation of neck pain is to be expected upon various movements, but is not diagnostic of any source of cause of pain.

- Testing passive, accessory, intersegmental movements has been found to be unreliable, and lacks validity.

- In patients with arterial dissection, examination of the neck will be normal.

Physical examination is a traditional component of medical practice. It is undertaken in order to obtain information that might assist in establishing or excluding a patho-anatomic diagnosis. Implicit in the conduct of physical examination is the belief that it is both reliable and valid. Assumption or assertion in this regard, however, does not constitute evidence. Just because someone believes or insists that a particular technique is reliable or is valid does not make it so. Not until the technique is subjected to formal scrutiny does evidence arise of its reliability and validity (see Chapter 25).

In many circles, physical examination of the musculoskeletal system is structured around the categories of inspection, palpation, and movement, sometimes summarized colloquially as: *look, feel, move*. Movement can be subdivided into active and passive physiological movements, and also into passive accessory movements.

(Physiological movements are those that a subject can execute themselves, i.e. the normal, obvious movements of a joint, such as flexion, extension, or rotation. Accessory movements are ones that cannot be executed in isolation by the subject, because muscles do not act in the appropriate direction. Typically they involve sliding or gliding movements of the joint, or rotations around the long axis of the joint. The anterior drawer test of the knee is an example from the appendicular skeleton. In the vertebral column, accessory movements include lateral gliding of the vertebrae, or forward gliding without rotation in the sagittal plane.)

In the context of the cervical spine, many of the traditional, and some of the more specialized, techniques of physical examination have been tested. Most investigations have focused on reliability. Few techniques have been assessed for validity.

GENERAL MEDICAL EXAMINATION

Certain tests that stem from general medical practice apply to the neck, and should be considered in the light of the patient's history and presentation. They are not explicitly musculoskeletal tests, nor have they been assessed for reliability and validity. However, they are accepted, and even hallowed, as classical signs of serious or visceral disorders that enter the differential diagnosis of a patient with neck pain.

Perhaps most striking in this regard is Kernig's sign. In a patient who is ill, with severe headache and neck pain, aggravation of pain by passive flexion of the neck is a hallowed sign of meningeal irritation, be that by blood in a patient with subarachnoid hemorrhage, or by inflammatory exudate in a patient with meningitis. The reliability and validity of this sign have not been questioned essentially because the diagnosis does not rest on this sign but is established by lumbar puncture.

Other tests include palpation of the viscera of the throat for masses and tenderness in a patient with anterior neck pain; and palpation of the lymph nodes of the neck for evidence of lymphadenopathy. Tenderness over the bifurcation of the common carotid artery has been considered a classic sign of carotidynia, but the specificity and utility of this sign has been questioned, as has the very existence of this condition.[1] Horner's syndrome can be a presenting feature of patients with dissection of the internal carotid artery.[2] Otherwise, however, the diagnosis of dissection of either the vertebral artery or the internal carotid artery rests on history and imaging. Conspicuously, bruits and tenderness have not been noted in the literature on patients with these conditions presenting with neck pain.[2,3,4]

In a patient with acute neck pain seen for the first time, or a patient with unremitting pain, the body temperature should be measured, since it is a simple test for infection. However, although fever is a highly specific sign of infection, it is not a sensitive sign. Fever occurs in only some 42% of patients with spinal infection.[5]

NEUROLOGICAL EXAMINATION

By definition, a full neurological examination is not indicated in the assessment of patients with neck pain. The common, and even the rare, causes of neck pain are not neurological disorders. For those reasons, a neurological examination is superfluous. It does not provide a diagnosis of neck pain.

Neurological examination is indicated only if the patient has neurological symptoms. In that event, however, the presentation is no longer that of a patient with neck pain but of a patient with neurological symptoms. If a patient with neck pain also has radiculopathy, a neurological examination is indicated not by the neck pain but by the radiculopathy. In that context, neurological examination is both reliable and valid,[6] but is beyond the province of this text.

For patients with neck pain but no neurological symptoms, although a full neurological examination is not indicated, practitioners may wish to satisfy themselves that the patient does not have an unnoticed neurological condition. For that purpose a screening examination would be reasonable. If the patient has no gross sensory loss or weakness in the upper limbs, and has been able to walk to the consultation, the chances are vanishingly small that a neurological disorder is the basis for their neck pain.

One exception to this rule pertains to patients with neck pain and headache. Under those circumstances it would be wise to perform fundoscopy to check for signs of raised intracranial pressure, in case the patient has a rare intracranial cause of neck pain (see Chapter 2).

The circumstances are different if the patient has been delivered to the consultation, as obtains after trauma. In that event, a careful neurological examination is warranted to "clear" the patient, i.e. to exclude neurological injury and to allow the patient to proceed to the next stage of assessment of a patient after trauma.[7]

INSPECTION

Inspection of the neck (and the rest of the body) may have general medical significance and some musculoskeletal significance. Inspection can reveal features such as a rash (related to spondylarthropathies) and pigmentation (related to neurofibromatosis), but these features pertain only to rare causes of neck pain. Inspection can reveal deformity, as in Klippel–Feil syndrome, but that observation does not necessarily indicate the cause of pain. A congenital deformity may be incidental to the actual cause of pain. Nor is torticollis a diagnostic sign. Its presence simply invites a consideration of the differential diagnosis of that condition (see Chapter 2).

There is no evidence that any postural abnormality is indicative, let alone diagnostic, of any cause of neck pain. No studies have shown that a forward chin posture, or a straight neck, is related to neck pain from any particular source or due to any particular cause. Recognizing a particular posture may serve to describe the patient but it is not a diagnostic test.

PALPATION

In a patient with neck pain, palpation of the cervical spine is essentially an exercise in finding tenderness. Furthermore, since the osseous elements of the cervical spine are largely inaccessible to palpation, palpation is mainly an exercise in finding tenderness in the posterior neck muscles.

The reliability of detecting tenderness in the neck muscles varies with the muscle examined, the nature of the patient, and the skills of the examiner. In one study,[8] reliability was good for palpation of trapezius and levator scapulae in subjects with no symptoms or only occasional symptoms of neck pain, but fell to unacceptable levels in the trapezius muscle in subjects with so-called disturbing symptoms (Table 6.1). (Disturbing symptoms included persistent pain and pain that interfered with activities.) Other studies have shown that the reliability of palpation of muscle tenderness over the neck and suprascapular areas varies from poor to fair (Table 6.2), but can be improved to good

values with closer attention to operational criteria (Table 6.3).

Palpation for tenderness overlying the articular pillars of the cervical zygapophysial joints appears to be a reasonably reliable test. It has a kappa score of 0.68, with a 95% confidence interval of 0.47 to 0.89.[11] The diagnostic significance of this sign, however, is not known. Its validity has not been tested. It is not known if tenderness in these regions implies a source of pain in the underlying joint or in the muscles overlying the joint. It has only been demonstrated that tenderness over the articular pillars distinguishes patients with neck pain from asymptomatic individuals.[12] In this regard, the sign has a sensitivity of 82% and a specificity of 79%, giving it a likelihood ratio of 3.9 (Table 6.4).

Table 6.2 Reliability of palpation for tenderness in selected muscles of the neck, in subjects with neck pain. Based on Viikari-Juntura[9]

Site of tenderness	Kappa
Upper spinous processes	0.47
Lower spinous processes	0.53
Right side of neck	0.24
Left side of neck	na
Right suprascapular area	0.42
Left suprascapular area	0.44
Right scapular area	0.34
Left scapular area	0.56

na: prevalence too small to provide valid data

Table 6.1 Reliability of palpation for tenderness in selected muscles of the neck, in subjects with no or occasional symptoms (NOS) and in subjects with disturbing symptoms (DS) of neck pain. Based on Levoska et al.[8]

Site of tenderness	Kappa	
	NOS	DS
Right trapezius	0.62	0.22
Left trapezius	0.60	0.15
Right levator scapulae	0.54	0.52
Left levator scapulae	0.24	0.42

Table 6.3 Reliability of palpation for tenderness in selected muscles of the neck, in subjects with neck pain. Based on Andersen and Gaardboe[10]

Site of tenderness	Kappa
Right upper neck	0.71
Left upper neck	0.67
Right trapezius	0.72
Left trapezius	0.78
Right levator scapulae	0.58
Left levator scapulae	0.71

Table 6.4 The validity of palpation over the zygapophysial joints as a test for the presence of neck pain. Based on Sandmark and Nisell[12]

		Symptomatic		
Test		Yes	No	LR
ZJ tender	Positive	18	11	3.9
	Negative	4	42	

ZJ: zygapophysial joints
LR: likelihood ratio

All that these data show, however, is that patients with neck pain are likely to be tender over the zygapophysial joints. The basis for this tenderness is unknown.

A dolorimeter is a device designed to improve the reliability of the detection of tenderness by providing a quantitative reading of the pressure applied to any chosen point. A formal study[8] has verified that the reliability of a dolorimeter in the neck is good, but it has no validity in discriminating patients with disturbing symptoms of neck pain from those without disturbing symptoms. In that regard, it has a likelihood ratio of less than 2.0.[8]

Among chiropractors, palpation for tenderness and palpation for so-called "muscle" signs has been shown to have variable reliability, both with respect to region assessed and between different observers (Table 6.5).

Overall, the available evidence on palpation for tenderness in the neck indicates that reliability is fair to good on average, but varies between studies and over different sites of palpation. The validity of tenderness as a sign of neck pain is moderate, but it has no demonstrated validity in pinpointing a particular source of pain.

Table 6.5 Reliability between three observers (A, B, and C) on palpation for tenderness and finding "muscle" signs in selected regions of the neck. Based on De Boer et al.[13]

		Kappa scores		
Sign	Region	A vs B	A vs C	B vs C
Tenderness	C1–C3	0.08	0.48	0.38
	C4–C7	0.08	0.18	− 0.04
"Muscle"	C1–C3	0.22	0.24	0.01
	C4–C7	0.53	− 0.10	0.03

Trigger points

By definition, trigger points are pathological entities affecting muscle that are characterized, in the first instance, by tenderness. In full, the diagnostic criteria[14] are:

1. a tender spot in a muscle
2. associated with a palpable band in the muscle
3. reproduces the patient's pain and referred pain
4. elicits a jump sign in the patient
5. elicits a twitch response in the surrounding muscle.

All five criteria have to be satisfied in order to make the diagnosis.

Notwithstanding the applicability or otherwise of this diagnosis and its reliability with respect to muscles of the shoulder girdle, it cannot be legitimately be applied to muscles of the neck. Conspicuous in the source reference on this topic are descriptions of cervical trigger points that expressly excuse those trigger points from satisfying the prescribed criteria.[14] Specifically, "TP_1 feels like a large, deep, lumpy mass of muscle which must be pressed very firmly to elicit referred pain. This TP_1 is usually found a centimetre or two from the midline at the C4 or C5 level."[14] The description of this point and its location coincides with that of the C4–5 or C5–6 zygapophysial joint. Similarly, "TP_2 in semispinalis cervicis is not characterised by a palpable band...."[14] It is located over the C2–3 zygapophysial joint.[15] Moreover, the pain maps of these so-called trigger points coincide with the maps of referred pain from the zygapophysial joints.[15]

For these reasons it has been argued that so-called trigger points of the neck cannot be reliably differentiated from underlying tender zygapophysial joints.[15] Therefore, finding tender spots in the neck muscles is not tantamount to having identified trigger points. Thus, palpation does not constitute a valid means of making a diagnosis of cervical trigger points.

MOVEMENT

For the assessment of musculoskeletal disorders of the neck, assessing range of motion seems to be an essential, traditional component of physical examination, but ironically lacks any scientific basis. Measuring the range of motion of the neck, in any direction, may provide a description of the patient, and it may provide an objective measure of disability or response to treatment, but it has no bearing on diagnosis.

One study found that measuring range of motion has only poor reliability when assessed by visual inspection, but reliability is improved to acceptable levels if a goniometer is used.[16] Another study found good reliability between observers, but only for distinguishing limited from markedly limited movement.[9]

However, no studies have ever shown that a particular type of restriction or any degree of restriction implicates one source of pain more than another. There is, therefore, no validity of range of motion in the diagnosis of neck pain.

Some motion tests are considered positive if they reproduce the patient's pain, but their validity for a particular source or cause of pain has not been explored. These tests include rotation with over-pressure, flexion-extension, the foramen closure test, and the brachial plexus tension test.[12] Such studies as have been conducted have been limited to determining whether these tests are positive in patients with neck pain compared with those with no pain (Table 6.6). These studies show nothing more than that patients with neck pain are more likely than normal individuals to have neck pain produced by movements of the neck.

Segmental motion

In certain disciplines, it is believed that a diagnosis of neck pain can be made if passive intersegmental motion is palpated and assessed. These beliefs have been tested and found wanting.

In one study, a manual therapist was shown to be very accurate in diagnosing cervical zygapophysial joint pain by examination of passive accessory, intersegmental movements.[17] The features diagnostic of a painful zygapophysial joint were abnormal quality of joint movement, abnormal end-feel and reproduction of the patient's pain upon moving the joint. The results of this study, however, cannot be generalized, for they pertain only to the therapist tested. No studies have yet shown that other therapists are equally valid, or that manual examination techniques are reliable between therapists. Furthermore, a review of this study lamented how few control patients were included, and therefore found the data uncompelling.[18] Subsequent studies[19,20] found examination of passive accessory, intersegmental movements to be unreliable, with kappa scores of less than 0.40.

In the chiropractic literature, one study found the kappa score for detecting asymmetry of joint play was only 0.01.[21] For the detection of "fixation" of the atlanto-axial joint, one study found a kappa score of only 0.15.[22] Another study found it to vary between pairs of examiners but nonetheless to be generally poor (Table 6.6).[13] Reliability at mid-cervical levels was also very poor, but at C6–7 it was acceptable (Table 6.7).

In essence, the available evidence fails to substantiate that palpation of intersegmental motion is reliable. Its validity remains to be explored.

SYNOPSIS

Physical examination of the cervical spine seems to be undertaken on the basis of tradition or habit. Although some tests have reasonable reliability, others do not. No test has been shown to have validity. One can, therefore, wonder why patients with neck pain should be examined.

The justification cannot be that it is necessary or helpful in formulating a diagnosis. The lack of reliability and validity deny that utility. However, this lack of justification does not constitute grounds for totally abandoning physical examination of the neck.

There are social grounds for physical examination. The patients expect it, and performing it communicates concern and competence to the patient. Conversely, not

Table 6.6 The validity of selected tests of neck pain. Based on Sandmark and Nisell.[12] The likelihood ratio for rotation with over-pressure could not be calculated because of the zero value

		Symptomatic		
Test		Yes	No	LR
Rotation + over-pressure	Positive	2	0	
	Negative	20	53	
Flex-extend	Positive	6	5	2.9
	Negative	16	48	
Foramen closure	Positive	17	4	10.3
	Negative	5	49	
Tension test	Positive	17	3	13.7
	Negative	5	50	

LR: likelihood ratio

Table 6.7 Reliability between three observers (A, B, and C) for detecting "fixation" at selected levels of the neck. Based on De Boer et al.[13]

		Kappa scores		
Sign	Region	A vs B	A vs C	B vs C
Fixation	C1–C2	0.23	0.09	− 0.03
	C3–C5	0.01	0.02	0.05
	C6–C7	0.40	0.45	0.41

performing an examination risks communicating disdain or neglect.

For diagnostic purposes, physical examination lacks validity. The only validity of physical examination pertains to distinguishing patients with and without neck pain. Patients with neck pain have tenderness and restricted movements that are not evident in asymptomatic individuals.[12] In a positive sense, therefore, physical examination serves only to find that patients have signs consistent with a complaint of pain. It does not establish the cause of that pain. This relationship, however, can be used in reverse.

It should seem very unusual for a patient with neck pain *not to have* tenderness or painful movements. In such a patient, a sinister or occult cause of pain should be considered. In particular, the literature is quite clear that patients with artery dissections as the cause of their neck pain conspicuously lack tenderness or aggravation of their pain by neck movements.[4] In such patients, the history should be carefully reviewed to seek clues for a vascular or other non-musculoskeletal cause of their pain.

IMPLICATIONS

Having obtained a history, the practitioner *should* perform a physical examination. That examination, however, should not be conducted with the intention or expectation of establishing a diagnosis. It should be undertaken in a manner that conveys concern and interest. It should look for tenderness and restricted range of movements. If these features are present, they can be taken as corroborating a complaint of neck pain. If, however, physical features are absent, the possibility of a non-musculoskeletal cause of pain should be carefully considered.

References

1. Biousse V, D'Anglejan-Chatillon J, Massiou H, Bousser MG. Head pain in non-traumatic carotid artery dissection: a series of 65 patients. Cephalalgia 1994; 14: 33–36.
2. Biousse V, D'Anglejan-Chatillon J, Massiou H, Bousser MG. Head pain in non-traumatic carotid artery dissection: a series of 65 patients. Cephalalgia 1994; 14: 33–36.
3. Silbert PL, Makri B, Schievink WI. Headache and neck pain in spontaneous internal carotid and vertebral artery dissections. Neurology 1995; 45: 1517–1522.
4. Sturzenegger M. Headache and neck pain: the warning symptoms of vertebral artery dissection. Headache 1994; 34: 187–193.
5. Goodman BW. Neck pain. Primary Care 1988; 15: 689–708.
6. Bogduk N. Medical Management of Acute Cervical Radicular Pain: An Evidence-Based Approach. Newcastle Bone and Joint Institute, Newcastle, 1999; 35–50.
7. An HS. Cervical spine trauma. Spine 1998; 23: 2713–2729.
8. Levoska S, Keinanen-Kiukaanniemi S, Bloigu R. Repeatability of measurement of tenderness in the neck-shoulder region by a dolorimeter and manual palpation. Clin J Pain 1993; 9: 229–235.
9. Viikari-Juntura E. Interexaminer reliability of observations in physical examinations of the neck. Phys Ther 1987; 67: 1526–1532.
10. Andersen JH, Gaardboe O. Musculoskeletal disorders of the neck and upper limb among sewing machine operators: a clinical investigation. Am J Ind Med 1993; 24: 689–700.
11. Hubka MJ, Phelan SP. Interexaminer reliability of palpation for cervical spine tenderness. J Manip Physiol Ther 1994; 17: 591–595.
12. Sandmark H, Nisell R. Validity of five common manual neck pain provoking tests. Scand J Rehab Med 1995; 27: 131–136.
13. De Boer KF, Harman R, Tuttle CD, Wallace H. Reliability study of detection of somatic dysfunctions in the cervical spine. J Manip Physiol Ther 1985; 8: 9–16.
14. Travell JG, Simons DG. Myofascial Pain and Dysfunction: The Trigger Point Manual. Williams and Wilkins, Baltimore, 1993: 312.
15. Bogduk N, Simons DG. Neck pain: joint pain or trigger points. In: Vaeroy H, Merskey H (eds). Progress in Fibromyalgia and Myofascial Pain. Elsevier, Amsterdam, 1993: 267–273.
16. Youdas JW, Carey JR, Garrett TR. Reliability of measurements of cervical spine range of motion: comparison of three methods. Phys Ther 1991; 71: 98–106.
17. Jull G, Bogduk N, Marsland A. The accuracy of manual diagnosis for cervical zygapophysial joint pain syndromes. Med J Aust 1988; 148: 233–236.
18. Gross AR, Aker PD, Quartly C. Manual therapy in the treatment of neck pain. Rheum Dis Clin North Am 1996; 22: 579–598.
19. Fjellner A, Bexander C, Faleij R, Strender LE. Interexaminer reliability in physical examination of the cervical spine. J Manip Physiol Ther 1999; 22: 511–516.
20. Smedmark V, Wallin M, Arvidsson I. Inter-examiner reliability in assessing passive intervertebral motion of the cervical spine. Man Ther 2000; 5: 97–101.
21. Nansel DD, Peneff AL, Jansen RD, Cooperstein R. Interexaminer concordance in detecting joint-play asymmetries in the cervical spines of otherwise asymptomatic subjects. J Manip Physiol Ther 1989; 12: 428–433.
22. Mior SA, King RS, McGregor M, Bernard M. Intra and interexaminer reliability of motion palpation in the cervical spine. J Can Chiro Ass 1985; 29: 195–198.

Acute neck pain: imaging

KEY POINTS

- In patients with neck pain with no history of trauma, no neurological signs, and no history or clinical indications of infection or malignancy, *there is no indication for cervical spine radiography.*

- In patients with a history of trauma, *cervical spine radiography should be undertaken in accordance with the Canadian C-spine rule.*

- If adequately performed, an AP, a lateral, and an open-mouth view are sufficient as a screening test for fractures.

- There is no indication for the use of CT as a primary screening test in patients with uncomplicated neck pain.

- CT is indicated only if plain films reveal or suggest a possible fracture that requires better resolution.

- SPECT scanning has a potential role in the detection of small fractures in patients with acute neck pain.

- There is no indication for the use of MRI as a primary screening test in patients with uncomplicated neck pain.

The short synopsis of this chapter on medical imaging is that, fundamentally, radiography is not indicated for acute neck pain. There is nothing that radiography is likely to show that is diagnostic of the cause of neck pain or its source. Nor is there anything that computerized tomography (CT) or magnetic resonance imaging (MRI) will show.

Medical imaging is indicated only if the history reveals clues as to a possible serious cause of pain that might be demonstrated by imaging. In that event, it is not the neck pain that constitutes the indication for imaging but the particular clue obtained from the history. If such clues are lacking, medical imaging is simply not indicated.

Nor is imaging indicated simply because the patient has a history of trauma. If the patient presents with neck pain after trauma, the Canadian C-spine rule applies (Figure 7.1, see following page).[1] According to this rule, radiography is predicated on three basic questions:

1. Does the patient have high-risk factors that mandate radiography?
2. Does the patient have any low-risk factors that allow safe assessment of range of motion?
3. Can the patient rotate 45° to the left and right?

As shown in Figure 7.1, different answers to these questions dictate whether or not the patient should undergo radiography.

In the light of this synopsis, readers who are content to accept the recommendation against medical imaging for acute neck pain, need read no further in this chapter. They can proceed to the chapters on treatment. Readers concerned about the proscription of medical imaging can read on, in order to appreciate the evidence that supports the proscription of imaging.

REFERENCE

1. Stiell IG, Wells GA, Vandemheen KL et al. The Canadian C-spine rule for radiography in alert and stable trauma patients. JAMA 2001; 286: 1841–1848.

PRINCIPLES

In the interests of good practice, not just evidence-based medicine, the question that should be answered is, why undertake imaging at all? Fundamental to answering this question is an understanding of what imaging can, and cannot, show.

Plain radiography has the ability to demonstrate the silhouettes of the cervical vertebrae and to provide some limited impression of the status of the joints of the neck. Its utility in the investigation of neck pain, therefore, is restricted to finding lesions that affect bone, but is limited by its sensitivity and specificity for these lesions. With respect to disorders of joints, its utility depends on the validity of the features that radiography can reveal as signs of joint pain.

Plain radiography can demonstrate fractures of the cervical spine, changes in the joints, and some features of the late stages of infection and tumors. It is said to be useful for screening for so-called occult lesions of the spine. The evidence shows that changes in joints lack any diagnostic validity; if tumors or infections are suspected, other tests are better than plain radiography, and occult lesions are essentially a myth. For the pursuit of fractures, the Canadian C-spine rule applies.

CT scanning can provide axial views of the cervical vertebrae, and modern techniques can provide aesthetically appealing three-dimensional reconstructions of the spine. None of these images, however, has been demonstrated to be able to show causes of neck pain.

MRI offers the advantage that it can demonstrate soft tissues, such as the surrounding muscles of the cervical spine and the nerves enclosed within it. Of all the available imaging tests, MRI has the best sensitivity and specificity for lesions such as infections and tumors, but these conditions are rare. For common neck pain, MRI provides no diagnostic information.

INFECTIONS

The most important point is that infections are a rare cause of neck pain (see Chapter 2). Taking an X-ray just in case the patient has an infection is tantamount to ordering a test that one can virtually guarantee will be negative. Imaging in the pursuit of infection is justified only if there are clinical cues of an infection being present, or risk factors for an infection (see Chapter 5). Yet even then, plain radiography is not the optimal investigation. If taken too early in the course of osteomyelitis or discitis, plain films will be normal, and the negative result will provide a false sense of reassurance. Plain films are diagnostic only once there has been substantial destruction of bone, which may be 3–6 weeks after onset.[1] Furthermore, not all spinal infections involve the vertebrae. In patients with epidural abscesses, only 44% show bone involvement.[2]

However, there is an imperative to diagnose infection rapidly, since spinal infection threatens the spinal cord; in one series, only 39% of patients made a neurological recovery for lack of earlier diagnosis.[3] For early diagnosis, plain radiography is not the investigation of choice. For the detection of infection, bone scanning and MRI are both very sensitive,[1,4,5] but MRI offers the advantages of better assessment of intervertebral discs and paravertebral soft tissues.[4] These qualities, however, do not justify the wholesale application of bone scanning or MRI as screening tests for neck pain. Their use is justified only when the patient has risk factors or clinical signs of infection, or when a blood count reveals leukocytosis or a raised sedimentation rate.

REFERENCES

1. Goodman BW. Neck pain. Primary Care 1988; 15: 689–708.
2. Darouiche RO, Hamill RJ, Greenberg SB, Weathers SW, Muscher DM. Bacterial spinal epidural abscess: review of 43 cases and literature survey. Medicine 1992; 71: 369–385.
3. Danner RL, Hartman RJ. Update of spinal epidural abscess: 35 cases and review of literature. Rev Infect Dis 1987; 9: 265–274.
4. Bassett LW. Magnetic resonance imaging in musculoskeletal disorders. Bull Rheum Dis 1987; 37: 1–6.
5. Berquist TH, Brown ML, Fitzgerald RH, May GR. Magnetic resonance imaging: application in musculoskeletal infection. Mag Res Imag 1985; 3: 219–230.

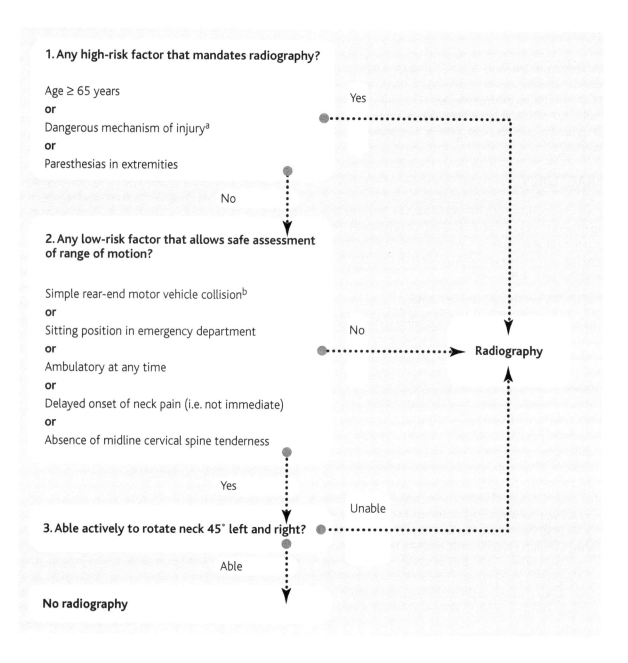

1. Any high-risk factor that mandates radiography?

Age ≥ 65 years

or

Dangerous mechanism of injury[a]

or

Paresthesias in extremities

Yes

No

2. Any low-risk factor that allows safe assessment of range of motion?

Simple rear-end motor vehicle collision[b]

or

Sitting position in emergency department

or

Ambulatory at any time

or

Delayed onset of neck pain (i.e. not immediate)

or

Absence of midline cervical spine tenderness

No

Radiography

Yes

Unable

3. Able actively to rotate neck 45° left and right?

Able

No radiography

a: Dangerous mechanisms

· fall from ≥ 1 meter or 5 stairs
· axial load to head, e.g. diving
· high-speed motor vehicle collision (>100 kph), rollover, ejection
· motorized recreational vehicles
· bicycle collision

b: Simple rear-end motor vehicle collision **excludes**

· pushed into oncoming traffic
· hit by bus or large truck
· rollover
· hit by high-speed vehicle

Figure 7.1 The Canadian C-spine rule.[1]

TUMORS

Similar considerations apply to suspected tumors. Tumors are rare causes of neck pain (see Chapter 2). They will not be evident on plain films early in their evolution. MRI and bone scanning are more sensitive at detecting tumors, and MRI is the most specific investigation.

FRACTURES

Even in patients with a history of trauma, fractures are an uncommon cause of neck pain (see Chapter 2). The problem that obtains is – when are plain films justified if a fracture is a possibility? Many authorities have wrestled with this question.

PATIENTS WITH NO SYMPTOMS

The emergency medicine literature offers certain guidelines as to when radiography is *not* necessary. The one finding that has consistently emerged from prospective and retrospective studies is that in *an alert and otherwise competent patient who has no neurological signs and who has no symptoms of neck pain* the chances of them harboring a cervical fracture is reportedly nil.[1-8] These studies have concluded that, in such patients, cervical spine radiography is not indicated. However, even though hundreds of patients were examined in these studies, calculation of the 95% confidence intervals reveals that even the largest study cannot confidently exclude a possible prevalence of fracture in such patients of 1%. At best, therefore, it can be concluded that in such patients fractures are extremely unlikely, but not impossible. Nevertheless, the American College of Radiology resolved that in asymptomatic, alert patients with normal physical examination radiographs were not necessary.[9]

These principles have been elaborated and tested in a prospective, observational survey of 34 069 patients in 21 centers in the United States.[10] Five criteria were applied (Box 7.1) which, if satisfied, required that the patient should not have cervical spine radiography. The survey found that these criteria had a sensitivity of 99.6%, and a negative predictive value of 99.9% (with 95% confidence intervals of 99.8–100%). Under the criteria, only two patients with clinically significant fractures would not have been detected had the criteria been applied. One of these patients had only an avulsion fracture of a vertebral endplate, which was asymptomatic. The other had a fracture of the lamina of C6.

One reason why physicians have undertaken radiography in patients with no symptoms has been the fear of occult cervical fractures. There have been several case-reports of patients with cervical fractures who

ostensibly lacked symptoms.[11-19] However, discussions of this literature disclose that either insufficient clinical data were provided in these reports or that, upon close scrutiny of the data, the patients had tenderness though no pain, or had been intoxicated (and were therefore questionably reliable), or in fact did have pain.[1,4,20,21] The one case that emphatically had no symptoms of neck pain was a patient with bilateral fractures of the femur and chest injuries.[16] The resolution among leading authorities is that in a genuinely asymptomatic patient, undistracted by other injuries, and who is alert and mentally competent, there is no risk of occult fracture.[4,21]

PATIENTS WITH SYMPTOMS

Of the clinical features that have been studied as putative signs of fracture, immediate onset of pain, midline cervical tenderness and impaired range of motion are very sensitive but only marginally or poorly specific (Table 7.1). These features, therefore, have only marginally useful likelihood ratios. Neurological signs and loss of consciousness have a high specificity and much higher likelihood ratios, but these are still far too small to overcome the low pre-test probability of cervical fractures.

Neck spasm, tenderness and neck discomfort are very sensitive features for fractures,[23,24] but lack specificity. The vast majority of patients with neck pain, tenderness and discomfort after injury do not have fractures.[3,24]

What is quite clear from the literature is that physicians are unable validly to predict from clinical features if a patient will have a cervical fracture. The large number of patients without fractures provides for good specificity, but the low prevalence of fractures despite clinical features impairs sensitivity. A formal study[23] determined that clinical impression had a specificity of 0.92 but a sensitivity of only 0.50 for predicting the presence of a fracture, and a specificity of 0.94 and a sensitivity of only 0.46 for predicting the result

Table 7.1 The validity of clinical signs as indicators of radiographically evident cervical spine fractures in patients with suspected neck injury. Based on McNamara[22]

Feature	Present?	Fracture present? Yes	No	Sens	Spec	LR
Immediate onset of pain	Yes	7	119	1.00	0.65	2.9
	No	0	225			
Midline tenderness	Yes	5	176	1.00	0.48	1.9
	No	0	164			
Impaired range of motion	Yes	2	137	1.00	0.60	2.5
	No	0	204			
Neurologic signs	Yes	1	7	0.14	0.98	7.0
	No	6	319			
Head injury	Yes	6	102	0.86	0.70	2.9
	No	1	239			
Loss of consciousness	Yes	5	21	0.71	0.94	11.8
	No	2	318			
Neurologic symptoms	Yes	0	36	0.00	0.89	0.00
	No	7	305			

Sens: sensitivity
Spec: specificity
LR: positive likelihood ratio

of the radiograph. In effect, when physicians expect that a patient will have a fracture, their performance is no better than guessing, or tossing a coin.

Neurological symptoms do not necessarily imply fracture. Only about one out of eight patients with neurological signs proves to have a fracture.[22] Neurological symptoms, however, are not universal; some 52% of patients with cervical spine injuries have no neurological signs.[25]

Nor is plain radiography a totally valid screening tool for fractures of the cervical spine. Single cross-table lateral views have been shown to be insensitive for the detection of fractures.[26–29] The types of fractures missed by single, lateral views are fractures of the odontoid, the lateral masses, laminae, transverse processes and vertebral endplates.[26] Of the unstable fractures missed on cross-table lateral, virtually all have been at the C1 or C2 level.[26]

Because of the insensitivity of cross-table laterals, the protocol recommended in the literature requires at least a lateral view, an antero-posterior view, and an open mouth view.[9,30,31] Whether or not oblique views should be added remains controversial. Some advocate adding oblique views in order to demonstrate certain fractures poorly evident on conventional three views,[32] but others have found no additional value.[33] Some have questioned

even the usefulness of the antero-posterior view, on the grounds that it reveals nothing not otherwise evident on the open mouth view.[34] The American College of Radiology reached no consensus on this matter.[9]

However, even a three-view series is not completely valid. Its sensitivity and specificity differ according to the findings on the plain films. Using tomography as the criterion standard, one study found plain films to overestimate fractures and underestimate the absence of fractures (Table 7.2).[26]

Another study using tomography confirmed fractures in only 14 of 55 patients with suspicious plain films, and detected undisclosed fractures in 13 patients; it found two fractures in three patients with reportedly normal plain films but with neurological signs.[35] In a small study using CT as the criterion standard, eight out of 13 patients with abnormal plain films were found not to have a fracture, but fractures were detected in four out of seven patients with normal plain radiographs, indicating a sensitivity of 0.56 and a specificity of 0.27 for plain films, and a likelihood ratio of on 0.78.[36]

A larger study, also using CT as the criterion standard, found fewer patients with missed fractures;[37] most were in patients with inadequate plain films, or films that showed suspicious features or overt instability;

Table 7.2 The validity of abnormal and suspicious three-view plain radiographs in the detection of fractures using tomography as the criterion standard. Based on Streitwieser et al.[26] Sensitivity, specificity, and the likelihood ratio have been calculated for abnormal and suspicious findings combined

Three-view radiographs	Tomography		Sens	Spec	LR
	Fracture	No fracture			
Abnormal	30	2			
Suspicious	5	5	0.92	0.71	3.2
Normal	3	17			

Sens: sensitivity
Spec: specificity
LR: positive likelihood ratio

no fractures were missed in patients with normal plain films.

Another study using CT confirmed fractures in 39 out of 54 patients with positive or suspicious plain films; found fractures in two patients with reportedly normal plain films; but found only one transverse process fracture in 123 patients with incomplete plain films.[38]

Reviews of this issue ascribe the imperfect validity of plain radiography in the detection of cervical fractures to inadequate exposure and position of the plain film,[39] poor quality of the radiographs and misinterpretation.[40] Such inadequacies can result in delays in diagnosis[40,41] and the risk of deterioration of neurological signs.[40] Nevertheless, it has been determined that if excellent, complete lateral visualization of the cervical spine is obtained, plus open-mouth and anteroposterior views, the risk of missing a significant fracture is less than 1%.[41]

Fear of missing a fracture (and being held culpable) is a strong motivation for ordering cervical spine films. Indeed, formal studies have found that "medicolegal purposes" is the single most common indication for cervical spine radiography.[42] A survey of physicians' attitudes revealed that 33% of all cervical spine studies are undertaken for medicolegal purposes, and more if the physician has previously been sued.[43] In another study, of 304 cervical spine studies, 236 were ordered for medicolegal reasons; yet only one fracture was detected.[42] The fear of missing a fracture is not justified by the epidemiological data.

Having distilled the literature and the expertise of its musculoskeletal task force, the American College of Radiology resolved that:[9]

- In patients who are alert and who have no physical signs of neck injury, radiography was not indicated.

- In patients with neurological signs or with symptoms of cervical injury, antero-posterior, lateral and open-mouth radiographs were indicated.
- In patients with an impaired sensorium, antero-posterior, lateral and open-mouth radiographs were indicated.

To these indications may be added the consideration that odontoid fractures are particularly common in the elderly.[30,44] Therefore, age becomes an indication for close scrutiny of C2.

However, while these guidelines go some way to rationalizing the use of radiography in the pursuit of fractures, they leave as ambiguous what constitute the "symptoms of cervical injury" that are an indication for cervical spine radiography. Almost any symptom might be interpreted as an indication. Nor are these guidelines of any help in dissuading physicians from ordering radiographs for medicolegal purposes, for they are not attended by statistical data that allay physicians' fears of missing a fracture.

REFERENCES

1. Roberge RJ, Wears RC, Kelly M et al. Selective application of cervical spine radiography in alert victims of blunt trauma: a prospective study. J Trauma 1988; 28: 784–788.
2. Fischer RP. Cervical radiographic evaluation of alert patients following blunt trauma. Ann Emerg Med 1984; 13: 905–907.
3. Kreipke DL, Gillespie KR, McCarthy MC, Mail JT, Lappas JC, Broadie TA. Reliability of indications for cervical spine films in trauma patients. J Trauma 1989; 29: 1438–1439.
4. Velmahos GC, Theodorou D, Tatevossian R et al. Radiographic cervical spine evaluation in the alert asymptomatic blunt trauma victim: much ado about nothing? J Trauma 1996; 40: 768–774.

5. Vandemark RM. Radiology of the cervical spine in trauma patients: practice pitfalls and recommendations for improving efficiency and communication. AJR 1990; 155: 465–472.

6. Roth BJ, Martin RR, Foley K, Barcia PJ, Kennedy P. Roentgenographic evaluation of the cervical spine: a selective approach. Arch Surg 1994; 129: 643–645.

7. Wales LR, Knopp RK, Morishima MS. Recommendations for evaluation of the acutely injured cervical spine: a clinical radiologic algorithm. Ann Emerg Med 1980; 9: 422–428.

8. Saddison D, Vanek VW, Racanelli JL. Clinical indications for cervical spine radiographs in alert trauma patients. Am Surg 1991; 57: 366–369.

9. Kathol MH. Cervical spine trauma: what is new? Radiol Clin North Am 1997; 35: 507–532.

10. Hoffman JF, Mower WR, Wolfson AB, Todd KH, Zucker MI, for the National Emergency X-radiography Utilization Study Group. Validity of a set of clinical criteria to rule out injury to the cervical spine in patients with blunt trauma. New Engl J Med 2000; 343: 94–99.

11. Thambyrajah K. Fracture of the cervical spine with minimal or no symptoms. Med J Malaya 1972; 26: 244–249.

12. Maull KI, Sachatello CR. Avoiding a pitfall in resuscitation: the painless cervical fracture. South Med J 1977; 70: 477–478.

13. Bresler MJ, Rich GH. Occult cervical spine fracture in an ambulatory patient. Ann Emerg Med 1982; 11: 440–442.

14. Walter J, Doris PE, Shaffer MA. Clinical presentation of patients with acute cervical spine injury. Ann Emerg Med 1984; 13: 512–515.

15. Haines JD. Occult cervical spine fractures. Postgrad Med 1986; 80: 73–74, 77.

16. Ogden W, Dunn JD. Cervical radiographic evaluation following blunt trauma. Ann Emerg Med 1986; 15: 604–605.

17. McKee TR, Tinkoff G, Rhodes M. Asymptomatic occult cervical spine fracture: case report and review of the literature. J Trauma 1990; 30: 623–626.

18. Mace SE. Unstable occult spine fracture. Ann Emerg Med 1991; 20: 1373–1375.

19. Mace SE. The unstable occult cervical spine fracture: a review. Am J Emerg Med 1992; 10: 136–142.

20. Mirvis SE, Diaconis JN, Chirico PA, Reiner BI, Joslyn JN, Militello P. Protocol-driven radiologic evaluation of suspected cervical spine injury: efficacy study. Radiology 1989; 170: 831–834.

21. Roberge RJ. Unstable occult cervical-spine fracture. Ann Emerg Med 1993; 22: 868.

22. McNamara RM. Post-traumatic neck pain: a prospective and follow-up study. Ann Emerg Med 1988; 17: 906–911.

23. Jacobs LM, Schwartz R. Prospective analysis of acute cervical spine injury: a methodology to predict injury. Ann Emerg Med 1986; 15: 44–49.

24. Roberge RJ, Wears RC. Evaluation of neck discomfort, neck tenderness, and neurologic deficits as indicators for radiography in blunt trauma victims. J Emerg Med 1992; 10: 539–544.

25. Gerrelts BD, Petersen EU, Mabry J, Petersen SR. Delayed diagnosis of cervical spine injuries. J Trauma 1991; 31: 1622–1626.

26. Streitwieser DR, Knopp R, Wales LR, Williams JL, Tonnemacher K. Accuracy of standard radiographic views in detecting cervical spine fractures. Ann Emerg Med 1983; 12: 538–542.

27. MacDonald RL, Schwartz ML, Mirich D, Sharkey PW, Nelson WR. Diagnosis of cervical spine injury in motor vehicle crash victims: how many X-rays are enough? J Trauma 1990; 30: 392–397.

28. Cohn SM. Lyle G, Linden CH, Lancey RA. Exclusion of cervical spine injury: a prospective study. J Trauma 1991; 31: 570–574

29. Lee C, Woodring JH. Sagittally oriented fractures of the lateral masses of the cervical vertebrae. J Trauma 1991; 31: 1638–1643.

30. Dreyzin V, Esses SI. Trauma of the cervical spine. Curr Opinion Orthop 1993; 4: 78–88.

31. Johnson DW. Imaging of the traumatized cervical spine. Curr Opinion Orthop 1996; 7: 61–68.

32. Turetsky DB, Vines FS, Clayan DA, Northup HM. Technique and use of supine oblique views in acute cervical spine trauma. Ann Emerg Med 1993; 22: 685–689.

33. Freemyer B, Knopp R, Piche J, Wales L, Williams J. Comparison of five-view and three-view cervical spine series in the evaluation of patients with cervical trauma. Ann Emerg Med 1989; 18: 818–821.

34. Holliman CJ, Mayer JS, Cook RT, Smith JS. Is the anteroposterior cervical spine radiograph necessary in initial trauma screening? Am J Emerg Med 1991; 9: 421–425.

35. Maravilla KR, Cooper PR, Sklar FH. The influence of thin-section tomography on the treatment of cervical spine injuries. Radiology 1978; 127: 131–139.

36. Mace SE. Emergency evaluation of cervical spine injuries: CT versus plain radiographs. Ann Emerg Med 1985; 14: 973–975.

37. Schleehauf K, Ross SE, Civil AD, Schwab CW. Computed tomography in the initial evaluation of the cervical spine. Ann Emerg Med 1989; 18: 815–817.

38. Borock EC, Gabram SGA, Jacobs LM, Murphy A. A prospective analysis of a two-year experience using computed tomography as an adjunct for cervical spine clearance. J Trauma 1991; 31: 1001–1006.

39. Acheson MB, Livingston RR, Richardson ML, Stimac GK. High-resolution CT scanning in the evaluation of cervical spine fractures: comparison with plain film examinations. AJR 1987; 148: 1179–1185.

40. El-Khoury GY, Kathol MH, Daniel WW. Imaging of acute injuries of the cervical spine: value of plain radiography, CT and MR imaging. AJR 1995; 164: 43–50.

41. Hoffman JR, Schriger DL, Mower W, Luo JS, Zucker M. Low-risk criteria for cervical-spine radiography in blunt trauma: a prospective study. Ann Emerg Med 1992; 21: 1454–1460.

42. Eliastam M, Rose E, Jone H, Kaplan E, Kaplan R, Seiver A. Utilization of diagnostic radiologic examinations in the emergency department of a teaching hospital. J Trauma 1980; 20: 61–66.

43. Miller RL, White S, McConnell C, Mueller C. Influence of medicolegal factors in the use of cervical spine and head computed tomographic examinations in an emergency setting. Emerg Radiol 1994; 1: 279–282.

44. Ryan MD, Henderson JJ. The epidemiology of fractures and fracture-dislocation of the cervical spine. Injury 1992; 23: 38–40.

CANADIAN C-SPINE RULE

Against this background, Canadian physicians developed a set of guidelines called the C-spine rule for radiography.[1] They apply it to trauma patients who are stable and alert. The rule operates as an algorithm, and is outlined in Figure 7.1. The rule respects and incorporates previous guidelines. It recognizes age as a risk factor. It recognizes neurological signs. It defines dangerous mechanisms of injury. The rule incorporates several factors that have been shown to be associated with low risk of fracture. These include some of the factors previously used to exclude radiography, but also cover certain "chestnuts" that have plagued this issue. In particular, being involved in a rear-end motor vehicle accident is included not as an indication for radiography but as a specific exclusion. The rule also recognizes that a patient who has been sitting or walking is unlikely to have a serious fracture.

The criterion standard for the rule was a serious fracture detected on standard three-view plain radiographs, i.e. AP and lateral, plus open-mouth view. Serious fractures were defined as all cervical spine injuries unless the patient was neurologically intact and had one of four injuries:

1. isolated avulsion fracture of an osteophyte
2. isolated fracture of a transverse process not involving a zygapophysial joint
3. isolated fracture of a spinous process not involving the lamina, or
4. simple compression fracture involving less than 25% of the vertebral body height.

When tested prospectively in 8924 patients, the C-spine rule achieved a sensitivity of 100% and a specificity of 42.5%. The lack of specificity of the rule meant that radiographs were still taken in 57.5% of patients who did not have fractures; but following the rule nevertheless resulted in an estimated decrease in use of radiographs of 15.5%. However, the high sensitivity meant that if the rule was followed, all clinical important fractures were detected; none were missed.

To physicians concerned about missing a fracture, the Canadian C-spine rule provides both solace and simple guidelines. The statistics are powerful, and provide assurance that fractures will not be missed, with a 95% confidence interval of 98–100%. The guidelines are simple and both easily memorized and readily implemented. Of particular value are the factors listed as indications for safe assessment of movement, such as able to sit, able to walk, and rear-end motor vehicle collision. These factors, however, should not be confused with indications for not taking radiographs. Patients who satisfy these criteria only qualify for the third step in the algorithm. Whether or not radiography is indicated is ultimately dictated by whether or not the patient can rotate 45°.

Perhaps most importantly, the Canadian C-spine rule is not a rule for all patients. It pertains only to patients who have a history of trauma and are alert and stable. For patients with obvious serious injuries, with multiple injuries, or who are not alert, radiography still remains indicated. On the other hand, for patients with neck pain who do not have a history of trauma, other guidelines apply (see below).

REFERENCE

1. Stiell IG, Wells GA, Vandemheen KL et al. The Canadian C-spine rule for radiography in alert and stable trauma patients. JAMA 2001; 286: 1841–1848.

FLEXION-EXTENSION VIEWS

For the patient with neck pain after trauma, some authorities have advocated flexion-extension views as a test for ligament damage.[1,2,3] These investigations have been endorsed by the American College of Radiology for symptomatic patients in whom ligamentous injury is suspected and whose plain films are normal.[4] Other authorities reserve this investigation for "high-risk" patients.[5]

As endorsed, these indications appear somewhat heuristic, in that a lesion (ligament injury) is presupposed and flexion-extension views are used to detect it. The literature could be misinterpreted as implying that flexion-extension views may be used in the search for the source of pain. Rather, flexion-extension views are a test of instability. They should be undertaken:

- in consultation with a spine specialist[5]
- if static plain films reveal markers or "fingerprints" of instability, viz.
  —kyphosis[1,5]
  —subluxation[1,5]
  —wedging of a disc-space[1]
  —facet displacement[1]
  —fanning of the spinous process[1]
- or if the patient exhibits
  —a neurologic defect or[5]
  —suffers inordinate neck pain[5]
- occasionally in patients with normal plain films who are considered at "high-risk" of having suffered a ligament disruption[5]
- only if and once the patient can perform movements under physician monitoring, which may be 10–14 days after injury[1,5]
- carefully, with small increments of movement[6] or under fluoroscopy.[7]

Notwithstanding these guidelines, a retrospective study found that the yield of flexion-extension radiographs was very low.[8] In 290 patients studied, flexion-extension radiographs revealed instability in only one, yet that patient had no symptoms at 1 month, and required no additional treatment. This study calculated that the 95% confidence interval for a positive finding of instability that required treatment was 0–1.3%. It also found that lack of movement, ostensibly because of pain, confounded flexion-extension radiography in some 34% of cases. The study recommended that flexion-extension radiographs not be used routinely. Instead, patients should be assessed clinically for the amplitude of movement possible. Patients without adequate movement could be evaluated at a later time, if indicated, when they were better able to flex and extend their cervical spine in order to achieve an adequate study.

REFERENCES

1. Fazl M, La Febvre J, Willinsky RA, Gertzbein S. Past traumatic ligamentous disruption of the cervical spine an easily overlooked diagnosis: presentation of three cases. Neurosurgery 1990; 26: 647–648.
2. Lewis LM, Docherty W, Ruoff BE, Fortney JP, Keltner RA, Britton P. Flexion extension views in the evaluation of cervical-spine injuries. Ann Emerg Med 1991; 20: 117–121.
3. Wilberger JE,, Maroon JC. Occult posttraumatic cervical ligamentous instability. J Spinal Disord 1990; 3: 156–161.
4. Kathol MH. Cervical spine trauma: what is new? Radiol Clin North Am 1997; 35: 507–532.
5. Vandemark RM. Radiology of the cervical spine in trauma patients: practice pitfalls and recommendations for improving efficiency and communication. AJR 1990; 155: 465–472.
6. Geisler FH. Comment on Fazl et al. Neurosurgery 1990; 26: 678.
7. Davis JW, Parks SN, Detlefs CL, Williams GG, Williams JL, Smith RW. Clearing the cervical spine in obtunded patients: the use of dynamic fluoroscopy. J Trauma 1995; 39: 435–438.
8. Wang JC, Hatch JD, Sandhu HS, Delamarter RB. Cervical flexion and extension radiographs of acutely injured patients. Clin Orthop 1999; 364: 111–116.

NO TRAUMA

A British study examined the X-ray findings and clinical history of 1263 patients studied at a single hospital over 12 months between July 1979 and June 1980.[1] The study included control cases referred for barium studies who did not have complaints referable to the neck. The results were striking and sobering (Table 7.3): *there were no unexpected findings of malignancy or infection in any of the films;* for which reason the authors concluded[1] that:

> *"the request for X ray films of the cervical spine 'just in case' such a finding is present is probably unjustified."*

What the study did find was a substantial prevalence of spondylosis. The prevalence of spondylosis increased with age, as did severe disc changes. Severe radiological changes in the zygapophysial joints were evident

Table 7.3 The prevalence of spondylosis and associated features in patients with and without neck symptoms attending a hospital radiology department over a 12-month period. Based on Heller et al.[1]

Age	N Case	N Control	Spondylosis (%) Case	Spondylosis (%) Control	Severe disc changes (%) Case	Severe disc changes (%) Control	Severe joint changes (%) Case	Severe joint changes (%) Control
Men								
< 40	63	29	21	10	6	3		
40–59	98	64	65	58	41	39	1	8
> 60	93	54	90	89	88	62	28	21
Women								
< 40	127	31	14	13	6	3		
40–59	166	98	58	56	39	29	7	5
> 60	106	89	85	88	79	61	16	21

only in the older age group. Spondylosis was more common in cases than in controls, but only marginally so; the difference was not of a magnitude to render spondylosis diagnostic.

Similar findings were obtained in an American study[2] that examined 1146 outpatient radiographic studies. Excluded from consideration were 85 cases of whiplash injuries, 69 bone surveys for known malignancy, 58 cases of known disease such as rheumatoid arthritis and disc herniation, 11 cases of follow-up after surgery, 6 patients with Down's syndrome, and sundry others, leaving 848 patients who underwent cervical spine radiography for vague, non-localizing, non-specific symptoms (Table 7.4). The study found that:

"In no patient was a serious diagnosis detected, including acute fractures, dislocations, or tumours."[2]

The findings were either normal, or other non-diagnostic features (Table 7.5).

The authors further found that on follow-up, only 12% of the population had continuing symptoms.[2] Moreover, follow-up data for as long as 5 years did not disclose any serious conditions that were missed on radiographs, which reinforced the authors' conclusion[2] that:

"…no medically dangerous diagnoses would have been missed if the cervical spine series had not been done."

Although no-one has formally reported the prevalence of serious conditions of the cervical spine in patients presenting with neck pain, the above-mentioned studies indirectly provide an estimate of that prevalence. Given that neither of these studies found any such condition and that each comprised about 1000 patients,

Table 7.5 Findings on cervical spine radiographs in patients with non-specific complaints. Based on Johnson and Lucas[2]

Finding	N	%
Degenerative changes	460	54
Normal	297	35
Muscle spasm	72	9
Congenital variants	9	1
Soft-tissue calcification	4	0.5
Old fracture	2	0.2
Miscellaneous	4	0.5
	848	100

with 95% confidence, the prevalence that such a large sample can exclude is 0.38%.

Thus, with respect to justifying cervical spine radiography "for fear of missing something", the prevalence of the conditions that underlie this fear is less than 4 in 1000. This means that a greatly disproportionate number of patients would undergo radiography in the attempt to find these elusive conditions. Accordingly, Heller et al.[1] recommend that:

"X-ray examination of the neck should be performed if there is a clinical suspicion of infection or malignancy or after some instances of trauma…

In most cases, however, there seems to be little point in requesting films of the neck to find cervical spondylosis."

CERVICAL SPONDYLOSIS

Cervical spondylosis is the single most common finding on cervical spine radiographs of patients with neck pain, rivalled only by a report of "normal cervical spine."[1,2] However, while it is a legitimate radiological observation, cervical spondylosis is not a diagnosis.

Individual radiographic features of cervical spondylosis occur with increasing frequency with increasing age in asymptomatic individuals[3,4] (Tables 7.6 and 7.7). This indicates that the features are age-related changes. Age changes most commonly affect the C5–6 and C6–7 segments, with those segments above and below these levels being progressively less commonly affected (Table 7.8).

In some studies cervical spondylosis occurs somewhat more commonly in symptomatic individuals than

Table 7.4 Indications used to obtain cervical spine radiographs. Based on Johnson and Lucas[2]

Indication	N	%
Neck pain or related symptoms	453	53
Upper limb pain, weakness	291	24
Headache	91	11
Back pain, weakness, numbness	65	8
Dizziness, blurred vision, hyperreflexia, chest pain	24	3
Lower limb pain, weakness, numbness	9	1
	933	100

Table 7.6 The number of asymptomatic subjects that exhibit features of spondylosis, by gender and age. Based on Gore et al.[3]

Feature	Men by age group (N = 20 in each group)				
	20–25	30–35	40–45	50–55	60–65
Narrowing	0	1	4	13	15
Sclerosis	0	1	1	10	13
Anterior osteophytes	1	5	7	16	19
Posterior osteophytes	0	1	4	10	14
Any of the above	1	5	7	16	19
	Women by age group (N = 20 in each group)				
Narrowing	0	2	6	9	13
Sclerosis	0	0	5	7	6
Anterior osteophytes	0	3	6	13	11
Posterior osteophytes	0	1	5	8	12
Any of the above	0	4	7	14	14
	Men and women by age group (N = 40 in each group)				
Narrowing	0	1	4	13	15
Sclerosis	0	1	1	10	13
Anterior osteophytes	1	5	7	16	19
Posterior osteophytes	0	1	4	10	14
Any of the above	1	5	7	16	19

Table 7.7 The prevalence of radiological features of the cervical spine in asymptomatic individuals. Based on Elias[4]

Feature	Number of subjects by age			
	< 30	30–40	40–50	> 50
Normal	24	18	18	2
Osteophytes	0	3	7	14
Narrowing of disc space	0	0	7	18
Sclerosis of articular surface	0	0	0	7
Osteoporosis	0	0	0	4
Calcification of anterior ligament	0	0	0	4
Loss of lordosis	0	0	0	4
Number of patients	24	21	32	25
Males:Females	5:19	7:14	20:12	18:7

Table 7.8 The prevalence (%) of age changes by segmental level in 160 asymptomatic individuals. Based on Fridenberg and Miller[5]

	Segmental level					
Feature	C2–3	C3–4	C4–5	C5–6	C6–7	C7–T1
Disc degeneration		7	13	30	26	3
Uncovertebral osteophytes	3	13	24	30	31	3
Foraminal encroachment	1	11	14	23	21	1
Zygapophysial osteoarthrosis	2	6	7	6	2	

in asymptomatic individuals,[1,6] but the odds ratios for disc degeneration or osteoarthrosis as predictors of neck pain are only 1.1 and 0.97, respectively, for women and 1.7 and 1.8 for men.[6] In other studies, the prevalence of disc degeneration, at individual segments of the neck, is not significantly different between symptomatic patients and asymptomatic controls.[5] Indeed, uncovertebral osteophytes and osteoarthrosis were found to be less prevalent in symptomatic individuals.[5]

Of significance is the false-positive impact of a report of cervical spondylosis. Such a report is more likely to lead to a referral to a hospital orthopedic department.[1] The reason for this is not evident, but presumably it is because of a belief that, somehow, spondylosis is diagnostic of neck pain and that orthopedic management is indicated. Yet, the evidence indicates that cervical spondylosis is not diagnostic of neck pain, and there is no evidence that orthopedic management for neck pain ascribed to cervical spondylosis is superior to any other management for neck pain.

REFERENCES

1. Heller CA, Stanley P, Lewis-Jones B, Heller RF. Value of X-ray examinations of the cervical spine. Brit Med J 1983; 287: 1276–1278.
2. Johnson MJ, Lucas GL. Value of cervical spine radiographs as a screening tool. Clin Orthop 1997; 340: 102–108.
3. Gore DR, Sepic SB, Gardner GM. Roentgenographic findings of the cervical spine in asymptomatic people. Spine 1986; 1: 521–524.
4. Elias F. Roentgen findings in the asymptomatic cervical spine. NY State J Med 1958; 58: 3300–3303.
5. Fridenberg ZB, Miller WT. Degenerative disc disease of the cervical spine. A comparative study of asymptomatic and symptomatic patients. J Bone Joint Surg Am 1963; 45A: 1171–1178.
6. Van der Donk J, Schouten JSAG, Passchier J, van Romunde LKJ, Valkenburg HA. The associations of neck pain with radiological abnormalities of the cervical spine and personality traits in a general population. J Rheumatol 1991; 18: 1884–1889.

LORDOSIS

Loss of lordosis is a feature sometimes reported in cervical spine films. This phenomenon, however, is a normal variant, and carries no diagnostic implication. It is equally prevalent among patients with acute neck pain, chronic neck pain, and no neck pain.[1] It is independent of age and symptoms but is more common in females.[1]

REFERENCE

1. Helliwell PS, Evans PF, Wright V. The straight cervical spine: does it indicate muscle spasm? J Bone Joint Surg 1994; 76B: 103–106.

CT SCANNING

Conspicuously absent from the literature on CT and the cervical spine is any recommendation that CT should be used as a primary investigation for neck with no neurological signs. If CT is used in this way in medical practice it is without any endorsement from the literature.

CT, and particularly CT myelography, has an endorsed utility for the investigation of radiculopathy and myelopathy,[1,2,3] but these conditions are not equivalent to, or synonymous with, neck pain (see Chapter 1). For the investigation of neck pain, recent textbooks specifically deny the use of CT for the investigation of neck pain,[4,5] there being no data to show any correlation between neck pain of any source and any feature evident on CT.

Where CT has an endorsed role is in the secondary investigation of patients with positive, suspicious, or incomplete plain radiographs of the neck, and in the investigation of patients with neurological signs. The latter is not pertinent to the consideration of neck pain, but the former is.

In this regard, some investigators have been liberal but ambiguous. One wrote: "CT scan should be obtained whenever cervical spine injuries are suspected, even when the standard radiographs appear normal,"[6] but this author did not provide a definition of the grounds for suspicion. Without specific indications, such prescriptions could be interpreted as justifying CT in every patient with a cervical injury, which is irresponsible given the rarity of cervical spine fractures, even among injured patients.

One study found the prevalence of fracture on CT in alert patients with no symptoms to be 1 in 138, the fracture detected being a fracture of the transverse process of C7.[7] Other studies have found CT to be of use only if plain films were positive or inadequate.[8,9] In the investigation with CT of patients in whom the C7 vertebra could not be clearly seen on plain films, the prevalence of fractures was 3 in 100, affecting the spinous process and lamina.[10] In patients with incomplete plain films the prevalence of fractures detected by CT was 1 in 123.[9]

One review described the utility of CT of the cervical spine, but prescribed its use only when plain films were positive, suspicious or inadequate; it reported that if plain films were adequate and unremarkable, the chances of finding a fracture were remote.[11] Another review recommended CT only if plain films were positive.[12]

Notwithstanding these general recommendations, two reviews have emphasized the utility of CT in assessing patients with suboccipital injuries, such as fractures of the occipital condyles and traumatic rotatory atlanto-axial dislocation,[13,14] as these conditions can escape detection on plain films. One study attests to an 8% prevalence of fractures of the occipital condyles, and C1 and C2 in severely injured patients.[15] The clinical guidelines for investigating the suboccipital region by CT include inadequate view of the odontoid on plain film, severe head injury, signs of lower cranial nerve injury, and pain and tenderness at the base of the occiput.[13]

In recognition of this literature, the American College of Radiology resolved that CT of the cervical spine was indicated:[14]

- in patients with neurologic signs or symptoms whose plain films are normal
- in patients whose screening films suggest injury at the occiput to C2 levels.

It recommended *against* CT in patients in whom ligament injury was suspected but whose plain films were normal.

SMALL FRACTURES

Tantalizing are reports that tomography or CT can detect small fractures that are not evident, or unlikely to be evident, on plain films. Such fractures include fractures of the lateral masses (articular pillars) of the zygapophysial joints or their facets.[16-20]

These fractures are noteworthy because they are difficult to detect, commonly overlooked, yet can be a source of pain. According to older studies, they occur in 3–11% of patients with cervical fractures,[21] but in studies using modern techniques their prevalence is of the order of 17%[19] or 20%.[17,18] Some 87% are not detected on plain films.[18] About one-third are associated with neurological signs[17,18] but the majority present only with pain.

Given that a large proportion of patients with chronic neck pain after whiplash injury suffered pain stemming from the zygapophysial joints,[22,23] it is tempting to try to identify articular injuries early. However, this does not justify speculative use of CT in the pursuit of what might be a rare lesion. Although facet fractures account for 20% of cervical fractures, the prevalence of cervical fractures after neck injury is only of the order of 2–4%.

Recommendations from those authors who have studied this problem include the use of CT or tomography:

- in patients with positive or suspicious findings on antero-posterior radiographs[16]
- in patients who develop radiculopathy[18]
- in patients with persistent pain.[19]

The last indication, however, is particularly vexatious because it does not take into account the low pre-test likelihood of the condition, and the risk of all patients with persistent neck pain undergoing CT. Moreover, in view of the radiation exposure involved, it is unreasonable to scan the entire cervical spine looking for a possible minute lesion. More efficient would be to screen patients with diagnostic blocks in order first to specify the likely level at which a fracture might be seen (see Chapter 13).

REFERENCES

1. Ellenberg MR, Honet JC, Treanor WJ. Cervical radiculopathy. Arch Phys Med Rehabil 1994; 75: 342–352.
2. Bernhardt M, Hynes RA, Blume HW, White AA. Current concepts review: cervical spondylotic myelopathy. J Bone Joint Surg 1993; 75A: 119–128.
3. Bell GR, Ross JS. Diagnosis of nerve root compression: myelography, computed tomography, and MRI. Orthop Clin North Am 1992; 23: 405–419.

4. Poletti SC, Handal JA. Degenerative disc disease of the cervical spine: degenerative cascade and the anterior approach. In: White AH (ed). Spine Care. Mosby, St Louis, 1995, 2: 1351–1357.

5. Barnsley L. Neck pain. In: Klippel JH Dieppe PA (eds). Rheumatology, 2nd edn. Mosby, London, 1998, 1: 4.1–4.12.

6. Mace SE. Emergency evaluation of cervical spine injuries: CT versus plain radiographs. Ann Emerg Med 1985; 14: 973–975.

7. Mirvis SE, Diaconis JN, Chirico PA, Reiner BI, Joslyn JN, Militello P. Protocol-driven radiologic evaluation of suspected cervical spine injury: efficacy study. Radiology 1989; 170: 831–834.

8. Gerrelts BD, Petersen EU, Mabry J, Petersen SR. Delayed diagnosis of cervical spine injuries. J Trauma 1991; 31: 1622–1626.

9. Borock EC, Gabram SGA, Jacobs LM, Murphy A. A prospective analysis of a two-year experience using computed tomography as an adjunct for cervical spine clearance. J Trauma 1991; 31: 1001–1006.

10. Tehranzadeh J, Bonk T, Ansari A, Mesgarzadeh M. Efficacy of limited CT for nonvisualized lower cervical spine in patients with blunt trauma. Skel Radiol 1994; 23: 349–352.

11. Acheson MB, Livingston RR, Richardson ML, Stimac GK. High-resolution CT scanning in the evaluation of cervical spine fractures: comparison with plain film examinations. AJR 1987; 148: 1179–1185.

12. Daffner RH. Evaluation of cervical vertebral injuries. Sem Roentgenol 1992; 27: 239–253.

13. El-Khoury GY, Kathol MH, Daniel WW. Imaging of acute injuries of the cervical spine: value of plain radiography, CT and MR imaging. AJR 1995; 164: 43–50.

14. Kathol MH. Cervical spine trauma: what is new? Radiol Clin North Am 1997; 35: 507–532.

15. Blacksin MF, Lee HJ. Frequency and significance of fractures of the upper cervical spine detected by CT in patients with severe neck trauma. AJR 1995; 165: 1201–1204.

16. Lee C, Woodring JH. Sagittally oriented fractures of the lateral masses of the cervical vertebrae. J Trauma 1991; 31: 1638–1643.

17. Clark CR, Igram CM, El-Khoury GY, Ehara S. Radiographic evaluation of cervical spine injuries. Spine 1988; 13: 742–747.

18. Woodring JH, Goldstein SJ. Fractures of the articular processes of the cervical spine. AJR 1982; 139: 341–344.

19. Binet EF, Moro JJ, Marangola JP, Hodge CJ. Cervical spine tomography in trauma. Spine 1977; 2: 163–172.

20. Yetkin Z, Osborn AG, Giles DS, Haughton VM. Uncovertebral and facet joint dislocations in cervical articular pillar fractures: CT evaluation. AJNR 1985; 6: 633–637.

21. Miller MD, Gehweiler JA, Martinez S, Charlton OP, Daffner RH. Significant new observations on cervical spine trauma. AJR 1978; 130: 659–663.

22. Barnsley L, Lord SM, Wallis BJ, Bogduk N. The prevalence of chronic cervical zygapophysial joint pain after whiplash. Spine 1995; 20: 20–26.

23. Lord S, Barnsley L, Wallis BJ, Bogduk N. Chronic cervical zygapophysial joint pain after whiplash: a placebo-controlled prevalence study. Spine 1996; 21: 1737–1745.

SPECT SCANNING

The issue of imaging patients with neck pain after trauma has been made more complicated by recent data on the utility of SPECT scanning. A small, but nonetheless alerting study has shown that SPECT scanning has the ability to reveal fractures and periosteal reactions to injury that were not evident on plain radiographs.[1] A retrospective review of 35 patients with neck pain following motor vehicle accidents, sporting injuries, and blunt head trauma compared what could be demonstrated on SPECT scanning with what had been seen on previous plain radiographs.

In 16 patients with normal cervical radiographs, SPECT revealed three with occult fractures. The nature of the fractures was not fully specified, but one example of a fracture of the lateral mass of C1 was illustrated.

In 10 patients with osteoarthrosis on cervical radiographs, SPECT revealed five with a fracture or post-traumatic arthropathy. The nature of the fractures was not fully specified but one example of a fracture of the lateral mass of C1 was illustrated.

In nine patients with a suspected fracture on plain radiographs, active fractures were excluded in six, and confirmed in two. The remaining patient exhibited non-specific activity.

The study implied that the fractures found were small and stable, for none of the patients exhibited neurological signs or deteriorated. At follow-up, 95% of the patients with normal SPECT scans had recovered by 6 months, but of those with an abnormal SPECT scan, 44% had continuing symptoms by the same time.

This study suggests that SPECT scanning could be a useful adjunct in the investigation of patients with neck pain after trauma because of its ability to demonstrate small, occult cervical fractures. In this regard, the authors recommend SPECT scanning between 2 and 6 weeks after the onset of pain, in patients with continuing symptoms.[1] Although finding a small fracture may not influence the patient's natural history, it has a putative bearing on management. Surgical management is not indicated for such small fractures, but immobilization may be preferable to physiotherapy. Indeed, it was the investigators' impression that those patients with fractures fared better when immobilized than when treated with physiotherapy.[1] Therefore, there appears to be a utility to using SPECT scanning in patients with post-traumatic neck pain. The added utility of SPECT scanning is that it can obviate the need for CT scanning in the pursuit of occult fractures. Instead of using CT to screen all levels of the neck for occult fractures, CT can be directed to a single joint found to be active on SPECT.

It is tempting to adopt the authors' recommended algorithm, in which SPECT scanning should be performed in patients with continuing neck pain at about 4 weeks, but given the small size of this initial study, this should be seen as a tentative recommendation. A larger study is required to determine more reliably the potential yield of SPECT scanning, and to determine if there are more specific clinical indicators that optimize the yield and prevent SPECT scanning becoming a routine investigation in any patient with neck pain after trauma.

REFERENCE

1. Seitz JP, Unguez CE, Corbus HF, Wooten WW. SPECT of the cervical spine in the evaluation of neck pain after trauma. Clin Nucl Med 1995; 20: 667–673.

MRI

There have been no studies of the utility of MRI in the investigation of uncomplicated neck pain. Such literature as is available pertains to the MRI features of the cervical spine in asymptomatic individuals and in patients with a history of whiplash.

The literature of cervical MRI in asymptomatic individuals provides conflicting but sobering information. Different studies do not agree on the actual prevalence of particular features, but they do agree that "classical" abnormalities are quite common, if not very common, in asymptomatic individuals[1,2] (Table 7.9).

This precludes invoking these abnormalities as causes of neck pain in symptomatic individuals.

There are no reports of diagnostic findings on MRI in patients with neck pain with no history of trauma or with no neurological signs. Thus, by definition, there is no indication for MRI for neck pain. Requesting MRI in such patients is tantamount to looking for entities that have not been described.

In patients with neck pain after whiplash, several studies have shown that MRI does not demonstrate any abnormalities consistent with, or diagnostic of, the cause or source of pain.[3,4,5,6,7] MRI reveals only those features evident in asymptomatic individuals.

The only positive report on cervical MRI relates to occult cervical spine injury in post-trauma patients.[8] Of 174 consecutive patients who had:

- a clinical history consistent with potential spinal instability, and
- equivocal cervical spine X-ray film, or
- equivocal physical examination, but
- no signs of myelopathy

62 (36%) were found to have disrupted discs or ligaments. The abnormalities found were considered to be of sufficient significance to alter management. This report is tantalizing in that it indicates that diagnostic abnormalities not evident on plain radiography can be seen on MRI, but it is frustrating in that it reports an incidence of abnormalities in patients with "a clinical history consistent with potent spinal instability."

Table 7.9 The prevalence of abnormalities on MRI of the cervical spine in asymptomatic individuals. Based on Boden et al.[1] and Teresi et al.[2]

Feature	Boden et al.[1] Age < 40 N = 167 Major	Minor	Boden et al.[1] Age > 40 N = 97 Major	Minor	Teresi et al.[2] Age > 45 N = 100
Herniated disc	3	4	1	4	
Bulging disc	0	5	1	5	44
Foraminal stenosis	3	4	9	14	
Disc narrowing	2	11	16	22	52
Degenerated disc	8		37		
Spondylosis	3	14	6	34	24
Cord impingement	9	9	1	18	27

At no time were the discriminating features of this history defined. Without such a definition the study cannot be reproduced, nor can its findings be generalized so that MRI might be used in a responsible manner.

Reviews of imaging for cervical spine injuries restrict the utility of MRI to patients with spinal cord injuries,[9] vertebral artery lesions,[9] and neurologic deficits.[10,11,12] No indications are specified for patients with uncomplicated neck pain.

REFERENCES

1. Boden SD, McCowin PR, Davis DG, Dina TS, Mark AS, Wiesel S. Abnormal magnetic-resonance scans of the cervical spine in asymptomatic subjects: a prospective investigation. J Bone Joint Surg Am 1990; 72A: 1178–1184.

2. Teresi LM, Lufkin RB, Reicher MA et al. Asymptomatic degenerative disk disease and spondylosis of the cervical spine: MR imaging. Radiology 1987; 164: 83–88.

3. Pettersson K, Hildingsson C, Toolanen G, Fagerlund M, Bjornebrink J. MRI and neurology in acute whiplash trauma. Acta Orthop Scand 1994; 65: 525–528.

4. Fagerlund M, Bjornebrink J, Pettersson K, Hildingsson C. MRI in acute phase of whiplash injury. Eur Radiol 1995; 5: 297–301.

5. Borchgrevink GE, Smevik O, Nordby A, Rinck PA, Stiules TC, Lereim I. MR imaging and radiography of patients with cervical hyperextension-flexion injuries after car accidents. Acta Radiol 1995; 36: 425–428.

6. Ronnen HR, de Korte PJ, Brink PRG, van der Bijl HJ, Tonino AJ, Franke CL. Acute whiplash injury: is there a role for MR imaging? A prospective study of 100 patients. Radiology 1996; 201: 93–96.

7. Voyvodic F, Dolinis J, Moore VM et al. MRI of car occupants with whiplash injury. Neuroradiology 1997; 39: 25–40.

8. Benzel EC, Hart BL, Ball PA, Baldwin NG, Orrison WW, Espinosa MC. Magnetic resonance imaging for the evaluation of patients with occult cervical spine injury. J Neurosurg 1996; 85: 824–829.

9. El-Khoury GY, Kathol MH, Daniel WW. Imaging of acute injuries of the cervical spine: value of plain radiography, CT and MR imaging. AJR 1995; 164: 43–50.

10. Daffner RH. Evaluation of cervical vertebral injuries. Sem Roentgenol 1992; 27: 239–253.

11. Bell GR, Ross JS. Diagnosis of nerve root compression: myelography, computed tomography, and MRI. Orthop Clin North Am 1992; 23: 405–419.

12. Kathol MH. Cervical spine trauma: what is new? Radiol Clin North Am 1997; 35: 507–532.

8

Acute neck pain: electrophysiological tests

KEY POINTS

Electrophysiological tests:

- serve no purpose in the investigation of neck pain
- are not indicated for neck pain.

For reasons unexplained, some practitioners are drawn to requesting electrophysiological tests for patients with neck pain, especially if they have referred pain into the upper limb. Seemingly they believe that performing nerve conduction studies or electromyography will help formulate a diagnosis. There are no grounds to justify such practices.

Electrophysiological tests detect abnormalities in nerve conduction. Neck pain does not involve such abnormalities. Patients with neck pain will not exhibit them. Consequently, electrophysiological tests will detect nothing, and are redundant.

There is not even justification for electrophysiological tests in patients in whom it is not clear whether they have somatic referred pain or radicular pain. In that context, electrophysiological tests do not detect or diagnose radicular pain.[1] Even for the assessment of radiculopathy, electrophysiological tests are no more instructive than a careful neurological examination.[1]

REFERENCE

1. Bogduk N. Medical Management of Acute Cervical Radicular Pain: An Evidence-Based Approach. Newcastle Bone and Joint Institute, Newcastle, 1999; 67–69.

Acute neck pain: algorithm for acute neck pain

In mathematics, equations are statements that describe the relationship between one or more variables. For some equations the value of a particular variable can be derived from a formula. That formula is a restatement of the equation in a form such that the desired value (i.e. the answer) can be calculated simply by substituting the values of other variables or constants. Some equations, however, cannot be solved in this manner. When more than one value remains unknown, there is no unique, or single, solution. Subject to variations in the values of other variables, any number of solutions might emerge. Those solutions, however, can be determined using an algorithm. An algorithm is a process, or set of instructions, that can be followed to provide a set of solutions in the face of different values of a set of governing variables.

There is no unique solution for the treatment of acute neck pain, no single treatment that should be used to generate the desired answer, namely the relief of pain. Each patient presents possibly with more than one variable, which variously may affect their response to more than one possible treatment. In order to obtain the desired solution an algorithmic approach is required. The algorithm accommodates various presenting variables and various interventions, with the objective of obtaining the optimal solution.

Figure 9.1 depicts an algorithm for the management of acute neck pain. The algorithm is designed to be practical. It describes actions that any, and every, practitioner *can* take. It does not involve esoteric procedures, nor does it require special training. The algorithm also reflects the best available evidence, but in two ways. Firstly, it incorporates interventions that *have been shown to effective*. Conversely, it omits interventions that have been shown *not to be effective*, or for which evidence of efficacy is lacking or less than compelling.

By omitting interventions that have not been proven, the algorithm is designed to discourage practitioners from perpetuating, or adopting, interventions of questionable value which cannot be relied upon to benefit the patient, and whose undisciplined use creates no more than an illusion of treatment. Rejecting that which is not effective is a measure designed not only to benefit the patient but also to render the practitioner more responsible professionally. By following the algorithm, practitioners can be assured that they are practicing according to the evidence, and not on the basis of hearsay, or out of desperation for something, or anything, that is supposed to work.

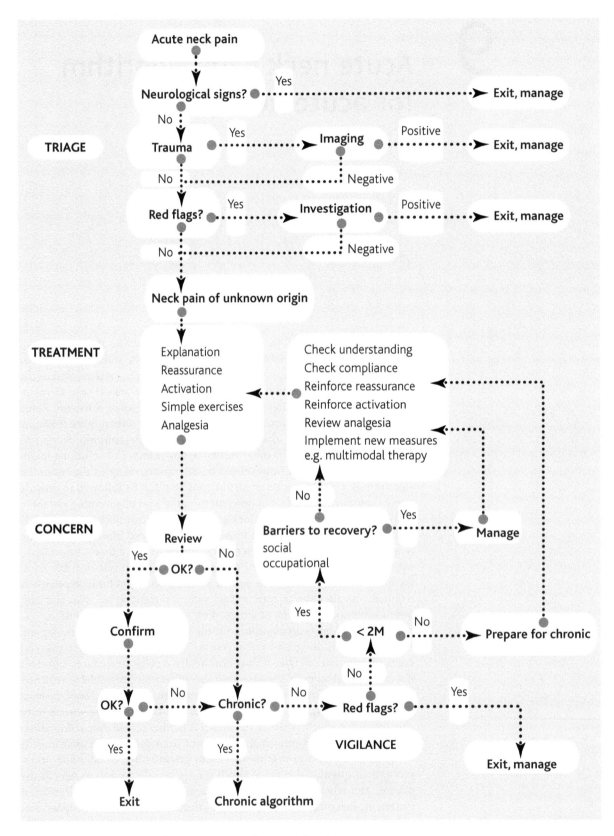

Figure 9.1 An algorithm for the management of acute neck pain.

This chapter is designed to explain the algorithm. In accordance with the theme of this section, the chapter describes what next should be done for the patient. The evidence and arguments that underpin the algorithm, and the reasons for selecting some interventions but omitting others, are described in the next chapter.

STRUCTURE

The core components of the algorithm are questions or actions, each depicted graphically as a box within Figure 9.1. For each question, binary responses are possible. Each response leads to a different, subsequent action or question.

The options are arranged in a spiral fashion, for the algorithm allows for two types of consequence. Either an endpoint is reached and the patient leaves the algorithm since it is no longer relevant to their problem, or the process recycles internally, in an effort to improve the status of the patient.

The various questions and actions are arranged into four domains, indicated in capital letters in Figure 9.1. Sequentially, these domains represent the four phases of management.

TRIAGE

Triage constitutes the initial phase of management. During this phase the practitioner should undertake an assessment of the patient, ostensibly to formulate a diagnosis. However, since it will be rarely possible to establish a patho-anatomic diagnosis, this process is largely an exercise of exclusion (Chapter 2).

The practitioner should determine whether the patient has any neurological symptoms or signs. If they do, they no longer qualify for management according to the algorithm. The patient converts from a patient with neck pain to a patient with a neurological disorder, and the management of the neurological disorder takes precedence over the management of neck pain. Management is continued according to established protocols for patients with spinal cord injury, myelopathy, or radiculopathy. If the patient does not have neurological signs, management resumes according to the algorithm.

If the patient has a history of neck pain precipitated by trauma they should undergo imaging according to the Canadian C-spine rule (Chapter 7). If imaging reveals a fracture, the patient no longer qualifies for management under the algorithm but is treated according to established protocols for fractures. If imaging reveals no fracture, management is resumed according to the algorithm.

The practitioner should carefully obtain a thorough history of the complaint (Chapter 5). The red flag checklist (Figure 9.2) can be used to screen for possible serious causes of neck pain. If grounds emerge for suspecting a serious cause, that should be pursued according to conventional practice for the disorder suspected. If the checklist denies any cues to a serious disorder, management can be resumed according to the checklist.

By the conclusion of the triage the practitioner will be in a position to formulate a diagnosis. However, a patho-anatomic diagnosis will not be available. Practitioners should not be distressed by the absence of this. They can be reassured that "no diagnosis" is what is to be expected for most cases of acute neck pain.

Name:				Neck pain		
D.O.B.				M.R.N.		
Trauma	Y	N	**Neurological**		**Endocrine**	
Fever	Y	N	Symptoms/signs	Y N	Corticosteroids	Y N
Night sweats	Y	N	Cerebrovascular	Y N	Diabetes	Y N
Recent surgery	Y	N	Vomiting	Y N	Hyperparathyroid	Y N
Catheterization	Y	N	**Cardiovascular**		**GIT**	
Venipuncture	Y	N	Risk factors	Y N	Dysphagia	Y N
Illicit drug use	Y	N	Anticoagulants	Y N	**Musculoskeletal**	
Immunosuppression	Y	N	**Urinary**		Pain elsewhere	Y N
Awkward posture	Y	N	UTI	Y N	**Skin**	
Manipulation	Y	N	Hematuria	Y N	Infections	Y N
History of cancer	Y	N	Retention	Y N	Rashes	Y N
Weight loss	Y	N	**Reproductive**		**Respiratory**	
Exotic exposure	Y	N	Uterine	Y N	Cough	Y N
(Overseas) travel	Y	N	Breast	Y N	**Signature:**	
Comments						
				Date:		

Figure 9.2 A checklist for red flag clinical indicators for neck pain, suitable for inclusion in medical records.

They should not feel obliged to be any more specific. They can rely on the evidence, which maintains firstly that no diagnosis is possible, and secondly that most traditional diagnoses are false (see Chapter 2).

Practitioners are, nevertheless, likely to want a label that they can use that reflects their having formulated a diagnosis. Technically, the patient has "neck pain of unknown origin," but this term is unwieldy and may not be satisfying either to the patient or the practitioner. Because the term contains the adjective "unknown," in the eyes of the patient it might imply failure or ignorance on the part of the practitioner. Instead, the practitioner can use one of two terms recommended by the Australian Acute Musculoskeletal Guidelines Group. For patients with no history of injury, the complaint can be called "idiopathic neck pain". For patients with neck pain after a motor vehicle accident, the label can be "whiplash-associated neck pain."

Practitioners should not be concerned if the patient appears dissatisfied with either of these rubrics. In the first instance, they are honest, and honestly reflect the state of knowledge about acute neck pain. They are preferable to false or erroneous labels, which may lead to inappropriate disease conviction or unnecessary alarm on the part of the patient. Secondly, any dissatisfaction constitutes a cue for one of the first steps of treatment. The dissatisfaction invites explanation.

Some practitioners may not be convinced by these recommendations. They may still prefer to use labels such as "soft-tissue injury" or "neck sprain," perhaps on the grounds that they are accustomed to doing so, or perhaps they find the terms more meaningful and more palatable to patients than "idiopathic neck pain." Part of the tension can be resolved by understanding the context of the arguments about taxonomy.

There is a difference between what practitioners think and write in their records and what they may say to their patients. The terms "soft-tissue injury" and "neck sprain" have no legitimacy as a diagnosis (Chapter 2). For that reason they should not be perpetuated in the professional arena. For recording a diagnosis, and for communicating that diagnosis, the terms "idiopathic neck pain" and "whiplash-associated neck pain" have been formally endorsed, and can be understood by fellow professionals. What practitioners say to their patients is another matter.

Practitioners might care to explain neck pain to patients in terms of soft-tissue injury or neck sprain, but explanation is not the same as diagnostic labeling. Labels should not be applied in a perfunctory or casual manner, particularly if they are false, illegitimate, or misleading. The priority is to explain the condition to the patient. Surrogate labels, therefore, constitute the beginning of an explanation, not a substitute for it.

TREATMENT

Two features characterize the initial phase of treatment. Firstly, it avoids all forms of *passive* treatment. Secondly, it concentrates on the patient's understanding, beliefs, and fears.

Passive treatment is avoided for two reasons. Ultimately, it is not effective, whereas other measures are (Chapter 10). More fundamentally, however, passive management is illogical. Passive management assumes that a specific diagnosis has been made of the source of pain and its pathology, and that the treatment to be applied will rectify that pathology. Neither assumption is true. No conventional examination or investigation can pinpoint the source of acute neck pain or its cause (Chapters 2, 5, 6, and 7). No conventional treatment has been shown to target any specific cause of pain or to be able to resolve it (Chapter 10).

Instead, a series of simple measures can be undertaken. To various extents, each has been shown to be as effective, or no less effective, than more elaborate interventions.

Explanation

Patients are unlikely to understand what the neck is and why it should hurt. They might not understand what neck pain means. They may attribute inappropriate significance to it, or harbor fears that neck pain predicates deterioration or spinal cord injury.

These possibilities do no invite a presumptive and perfunctory lecture on the anatomy and pathology of the cervical spine. Nevertheless, some form of explanation will be required.

One approach can be to couple explanation with reassurance (explained below). In doing so, the practitioner should remain alert to the patient's response, not only listening to what they say but also watching their body language for signs of confusion or dissatisfaction.

If required, another approach can be introduced. The practitioner can ask calmly:

"Why do you think your neck hurts," or

"What do you think is causing your pain."

If the patient reveals particular concerns or mistaken beliefs, these can be promptly addressed and corrected. If the patient reveals fears about serious causes or dire consequences, the practitioner can be confidently reassuring, for their assessment, to date, more than effectively rules out such conditions; and they can proceed to reassurance.

If the patient reveals no particular concerns, or responds:

"I don't know," or

"I don't know; you're the doctor,"

the practitioner can proceed by incorporating explanation into reassurance.

Reassurance

At his or her disposal, the practitioner has the evidence-base concerning the causes of neck pain (Chapter 2) and its natural history (Chapter 4). The fact is that serious causes of neck pain are rare, but can be recognized from the history. Meanwhile common causes are not serious and not threatening. Subsequently, the natural history of acute neck is favorable. Even without treatment, patients can expect to recover. Relating these facts to the patient constitutes evidence-based practice.

Different practitioners will have different styles of communication, and different patients may require adaptations of any core approach to explanation and reassurance. It is not possible to articulate one single approach suitable for every circumstance, but one model could be to say:

"[Patient's name], I have listened carefully to your story, and I have examined your neck. From what I have heard and from what I have felt, I am confident that you do not have any serious cause for your neck pain. There is nothing that suggests that either I or you should be concerned.

You are like many other people, around the world who develop neck pain, but research has shown us that serious causes are rare, and usually present with some clue other than just the pain. You do not have any of those clues. For that reason I can be confident, and you can be confident, that your neck pain does not have a serious cause. In the vast majority of cases, no one knows what causes the pain, but it is probably something simple, like a sprain or sore muscles. There is no simple way to make an exact diagnosis. But, at the same time, there is no need to do so. Research has shown that most people like you make a full recovery in due course, even without treatment.

In your case, we can rely on that. Our greatest tool is the passage of time. It is highly likely that this episode of pain will settle of its own accord. In the meantime, however, we are going to do a few things to help that process along."

In such a manner, the practitioner conveys to the patient the facts concerning cause and natural history. By deferring to research that shows that no one can make a diagnosis and that there is no need to do so, the practitioner avoids being seen as not knowing.

What is critical is that reassurance is not dismissive. It is probably true that, left untreated, the patient will recover; but that may not be satisfying to the patient. The closing paragraph of the reassurance states that the practitioner and patient can rely on natural history, but the patient will not be abandoned to it, in isolation. The practitioner closes the reassurance of the patient by leading into measures that both parties can take to improve on the natural history.

Activation

Maintaining activity as near to normal as possible is a critical measure in the early management of acute neck pain. It is of paramount importance in preventing unwarranted disability.

Three precepts apply. The practitioner must:

1. encourage and convince the patient to resume or maintain normal activities
2. identify any barriers to doing so
3. be prepared to suggest alternative means of maintaining activities if the patient's native way of doing them is impeded by the pain.

At the disposal of the practitioner is evidence that patients who do resume or maintain normal activities recover well, and in proportions better, or at least no worse, than in those who undergo passive treatments (see Chapter 10).

The patient may be apprehensive about resuming activities, or fearful that doing so will aggravate their pain. They may believe that rest is indicated. The response can include explanations to the effect that there is no injury to their neck that will be worsened by resuming activity, and no injury that requires rest. Indeed, it can be emphasized that rest is potentially deleterious; stiffness due to immobilization needs to be avoided; and the neck must be encouraged to heal in a manner that allows normal function in the future. Accordingly, resuming activities serves to remind the neck of what is expected of it. Meanwhile, if pain appears to be the only barrier to activity, other measures are about to be taken to deal with that issue.

It is not practical to catalogue all the things that patients might say they cannot do because of neck pain, or what alternatives might be entertained. Nor are there any specific ergonomic rules. In this context, the practitioner needs only to be attentive and creative. They can start by identifying a handful of key activities, in the first instance, that the patient expects not to be able to undertake. Once the key activities have been addressed, in subsequent consultations, if necessary, remaining problems can be systematically addressed.

In most instances, normal activities can be resumed despite the pain, and without any explicit measures. In some instances activities might need to be resumed by setting goals and progressing towards those goals in a planned and measured way. If sustained activities are barrier, those activities can be undertaken for short periods initially but progressing to increasingly longer periods.

Aggravation of pain, or fear of aggravation, is usually the alleged barrier in these circumstances. However, resumption of activities should not be brutal exercise. It is undertaken in the context of other interventions being undertaken to address the pain. Consequently, the patient can expect that as the pain is reduced—be that by natural history or by additional measures—their capacity for activity and endurance will improve. The vital measure is to avoid non-resumption of activity, and regression to disability.

Specific measures of an ergonomic nature might be required if certain activities legitimately and unavoidably aggravate the patient's pain. The principle at hand is not to cease the activity but to devise a means of maintaining it in a novel manner. The solutions rely on the practitioner's insights and creativity. The possibilities are virtually endless and cannot be listed, but some examples serve to underscore the principle.

- If deskwork aggravates the patient's pain because they have to look down, the solution is to raise the work so that they do not have to look down.
- If reversing a motor vehicle is a problem because the patient cannot rotate the head to the rear, learning how to use mirrors becomes a solution.
- If hanging *up* the washing aggravates the pain, measures might be taken to convert the task to hanging *down* the washing. Either the clothes line can be lowered to below shoulder height while the washing is pegged, or a box-platform can be used so that patient can stand taller than the clothes line.

Simple exercises

Exercises designed to keep the neck moving are perhaps the single most effective measure for the treatment of acute neck pain. They couple perfectly with the objective of resuming normal activities. In addition, they can be portrayed as a therapeutic measure in their own right. Most critically, they are something that the patient does him- or herself.

This latter feature serves two purposes. Firstly, patients have an intervention at their disposal that they can administer. They should do the exercises as an analgesic measure. This includes time-contingent administration and first aid. The patient should undertake the exercises at prescribed times, the objective being to keep the neck mobile and to increase range if it has been restricted. A suitable regimen is "at every ceremonial time of the day, i.e. on rising, at morning tea, at lunchtime, at afternoon tea, and in the evening; or before you start a task, and immediately after finishing the task." Between times, the exercises can be used as a preventive measure if the pain appears to threaten to "flare", or if a forthcoming activity threatens to aggravate the pain.

Secondly, patients avoid passive interventions and are personally empowered. They are given a means by which they become responsible for their own rehabilitation and recovery. Given something that they can do, on their own, they avoid becoming dependent on others to provide relief or to care for them; treatment can be applied whenever it is needed, wherever it is needed. It is not restricted by the availability of a therapist.

The exercises are not designed to treat any specific lesion. Indeed, they cannot be so, for no lesion can be diagnosed. Nor are they designed to increase strength or endurance. The objectives of the exercises are to increase and maintain mobility. For these purposes a variety of exercises have been described.[2,3] One source provides them in a form that the patient can take home and use.[4]

Practitioners who are able, and feel competent to do so, can themselves instruct patients in how to perform these exercises. A virtue of doing so is that, at follow-up consultations they can check the patient's understanding of the exercises and their compliance with them. If required, the practitioner can correct any misunderstandings and reinforce compliance. This facility is not possible if the practitioner does not know the exercises.

If required, the practitioner can enlist the assistance of a colleague in musculoskeletal medicine or physical therapy who can instruct the patient in the required exercises and monitor the patient's progress and compliance with them. In that event, however, the assistance lies in instructing the patient. It does not amount to discharging the patient to the care of another. It does not amount to referring the patient for "physiotherapy." The imperative is to instruct patients in exercises that empower them to be responsible for their own rehabilitation. That should not be confused, deliberately or inadvertently with referral for passive therapy. Therefore, the colleague that the practitioner enlists must be someone who understands the context of evidence-based practice for acute neck pain.

Analgesia

Providing analgesia is a vexatious issue. Practitioners will be drawn to providing the patient with something that relieves the pain, but evidence is lacking that any particular analgesic is effective for acute neck pain (Chapter 10).

On the basis of consensus only, the Australian Guidelines[1] recommend the use of paracetamol (USAN acetaminophen) if an analgesic is required. If practitioners prescribe paracetamol they should understand that it is only the basis of the reputation of this drug as an analgesic for other conditions, such as arthritis, dental and post-operative pain. Its efficacy for any form of spinal pain has not been demonstrated, and is probably no better than that of natural history.

If patients appear to require stronger analgesia, practitioners may be tempted to use other drugs. Compound analgesics (combinations of paracetamol and codeine) are not appropriate. They provide only marginally greater analgesia (5%) over paracetamol alone, but incur significantly more side-effects.[5] Nor have non-steroidal anti-inflammatory agents been shown to be more effective than paracetamol for neck pain (Chapter 10).

As a next step, the only option are opioids, but no studies have shown opioids to be effective for neck pain. The Australian Guidelines allow for opioids to be used for patients with severe acute neck pain, but they counsel also that, in such patients, careful consideration be given as to why the patient's pain is so severe. It may be that they require revised investigation for an undisclosed serious cause of pain. Any use of opioids should be closely monitored, lest features emerge of a previously undisclosed serious cause of pain. If none appear, other reasons for the severity of pain should be explored in consultation with a pain clinic.

CONCERN

Concern is possibly an unusual domain of management. Most practitioners might feel that their responsibilities are acquitted once they have assessed the patient and prescribed treatment. They may feel that they are too busy to afford additional consultations. Such a limited intervention, however, risks creating the illusion of success, and also risks abandoning patients both literally and figuratively.

Concern is the implicit effect of the third domain of management. The first explicit step is to review the patient. That review should be premeditated and scheduled. Patients who were distressed at the initial consultation should be reviewed soon: within 1, 2 or 3 days, depending on the practitioner's assessment of the degree of distress. Others can be reviewed in a week or so.

Review provides the opportunity for the practitioner to determine if the patient has recovered, or is recovering; or if they are not progressing. Deliberate review allows the practitioner to recognize if treatment is not succeeding. It also prevents patients from feeling abandoned.

If the patient is recovering, further review may not be required. Nevertheless, it seems wise to confirm that recovery has persisted, lest the patient has had a relapse. That confirmation may require no more than a telephone call, rather than a formal consultation. Such follow-up could be conducted by a practice assistant.

If the patient has not recovered, and is either not recovering or recovering too slowly, the review provides the opportunity to revisit treatment. Paramount at this stage is to check understanding and compliance. Patients may be not recovering because they did not fully understand what the practitioner said at the first consultation; they may not be undertaking assiduously the treatment that was prescribed. In that event, the review provides the opportunity to reinforce the earlier prescriptions.

If the earlier prescribed interventions have been followed correctly, the practitioner should judge if persisting with them might be sufficient. In that event a further review should be scheduled.

If the earlier prescribed interventions appear to be ineffective or insufficient, consideration can be given to implementing additional or alternative interventions. The leading option is multimodal therapy, which involves a combination of exercises guided by therapists and manual therapy (Chapter 10).

Meanwhile, if patients are not recovering, other barriers to recovery should be explored. These may be personal, social, or occupational. They can be discovered only by careful and sensitive enquiry. They may need to be explored in an indirect manner. The practitioner can enter the realm by pursuing general lines of enquiry such as:

"So, what else is happening in your life?" or

"How are things at work?"

If barriers are revealed, they may be amenable to correction. Depending on the circumstances of the practitioner, practitioners themselves may be able to intervene, or they may need to enlist the services of others, for example a counselor for personal problems, or an occupational physician for occupational matters.

By engaging this process of review, reinforcement, and exploration of additional issues, the practitioner will not abandon patients who are having difficulties recovering. In most cases, patients should recover under these conditions: some sooner, some later. However, it is inevitable that some patients will not recover. Their lack of response predicts that they will progress to persistent or chronic pain.

The algorithm asks that practitioners persist with the prescribed interventions for 2 months. If patients are going to recover, they will do so within this period,

Name:_____				Neck pain			
D.O.B._____				M.R.N._____			
▓▓▓▓▓▓			**Neurological**	▓▓▓▓▓▓▓▓			
Fever	Y	N	Symptoms/signs	Y	N		
Night sweats	Y	N	Cerebrovascular	Y	N		
			Vomiting	Y	N		
▓▓▓▓▓▓			▓▓▓▓▓▓	**GIT**			
▓▓▓▓▓▓			▓▓▓▓▓▓	Dysphagia		Y	N
▓▓▓▓▓▓			▓▓▓▓▓▓	**Musculoskeletal**			
▓▓▓▓▓▓			**Urinary**	Pain elsewhere		Y	N
▓▓▓▓▓▓			UTI	Y	N	**Skin**	
Manipulation	Y	N	Hematuria	Y	N	Infections	Y	N
			Retention	Y	N	Rashes	Y	N
Weight loss	Y	N	**Reproductive**			**Respiratory**	
▓▓▓▓▓▓			▓▓▓▓▓▓	Cough		Y	N
				Signature:			
Comments							
				Date:			

Figure 9.3 The checklist for red flag clinical indicators for neck pain, modified to delete items of past history but retaining domains relating to the development of new symptoms.

or they will show sufficient signs of recovery that persisting with the interventions is justified.

If, however, recovery is not evident, there seems little point in persisting until the patient reaches the statutory 3 months that would qualify them as having chronic pain. At about 2 months, preparations should be undertaken for how the patient is going to be managed in the event that their pain persists. The difference between 2 months and 3 months may be what is required to secure appointments with specialist services without inheriting too much decompensation of the patient.

VIGILANCE

Serious causes of neck pain may not present in a florid manner at the time that pain starts. Signs of a serious cause may not be evident on the occasion of the first consultation with the patient. Some serious causes may develop slowly.

Consequently, practitioners who see patients with acute neck pain should not be expected to make a diagnosis on the first occasion. Nor should they expect it of themselves. Not only is it unfair to expect this, it may not be biologically possible to do so.

That is not to say, however, that all responsibility ceases after the conclusion of the first triage. The practitioner should remain alert to the possibility of the later emergence of features of a potentially serious condition. Accordingly, the practitioner should remain vigilant to the appearance of new cues that might demand a reformulation of the working diagnosis.

Vigilance involves remembering to ask about new symptoms. The red flag checklist can be amended to serve as a recurrent prompt in this regard (Figure 9.3). Matters of past history no longer obtain; they will already have been recorded during triage. Vigilance requires attention to the emergence of new symptoms and signs.

By remaining vigilant, practitioners can be assured that they will not miss the emergence of a serious condition. By recording the absence of new symptoms on each occasion that they review patients, practitioners maintain evidence that they have not been negligent.

References

1. Australian Acute Musculoskeletal Pain Guidelines Group. Evidence-Based Management of Acute Musculoskeletal Pain. Australian Academic Press, Brisbane, 2003. (Online. Available at http://www.nhmrc.gov.au)
2. McKinney LA, Dornan JO, Ryan M. The role of physiotherapy in the management of acute neck sprains following road-traffic accidents. Arch Emergency Med 1989; 6: 27–33.
3. McKenzie RA. The Cervical and Thoracic Spine: Mechanical Diagnosis and Treatment. Spinal Publications, Waikanae, New Zealand, 1990.
4. McKenzie RA. Treat your own Neck. Spinal Publications, Waikanae, New Zealand, 1983.
5. de Craen AJ, Di Giulio G, Lampe-Schoenmaeckers JE, Kessels AG, Kleijnen J. Analgesic efficacy and safety of paracetamol-codeine combinations versus paracetamol alone: a systematic review. British Medical Journal 1996; 313: 321–325.

Acute neck pain: the evidence for treatment

As described in the algorithm for acute neck pain, certain interventions are recommended (Chapter 9). At the same time, other interventions are avoided or omitted. The basis for the inclusion or exclusion of interventions is the nature and strength of the published evidence concerning each.

EXPLANATION AND REASSURANCE

There happens to be no direct evidence of the efficacy of explanation and reassurance for the treatment of acute neck pain. However, this intervention was recommended by consensus by the Australian Acute Musculoskeletal Pain Guidelines Group.[1]

This recommendation has face validity, in that it makes sense to provide patients with an explanation of the condition that they are suffering. Furthermore, if reassurance is based on relating to the patient the data on the favorable natural history of neck pain, it becomes evidence-based practice. Confidence in the recommendation is enhanced by the knowledge that concerted explanation and reassurance has been shown to be effective in the management of acute low back pain.[2]

REFERENCES

1. Australian Acute Musculoskeletal Pain Guidelines Group. Evidence-Based Management of Acute Musculoskeletal Pain. Australian Academic Press, Brisbane, 2003. (Online. Available at http://www.nhmrc.gov.au/publications/synopses/cp94syn.htm)
2. McGuirk B, King W, Govind J, Lowry J, Bogduk N. The safety, efficacy, and cost-effectiveness of evidence-based guidelines for the management of acute low back pain in primary care. Spine 2001; 26: 2615–2622.

ACTIVATION

Several reviews and guidelines have recommended staying active as the core intervention for acute neck pain.[1,2,3,4] That recommendation, however, is based largely on the proven success of activation for the treatment of acute low back pain.[5]

Although activation has not been as extensively studied and reviewed as it has been for back pain, there is nevertheless some evidence for its efficacy in neck pain.

Two studies coupled "keeping the neck active" with exercise treatment.[6,7,8] To a large extent the data from those studies probably pertains to the efficacy of exercise. For that reason they are described in detail in the section on Exercises. However, the exercises were not designed to strengthen neck muscles or to increase their endurance, which has been the classical focus of exercise therapy. Instead they were designed to be a means by which patients themselves could keep their necks moving. To that extent, therefore, the studies provide support for the virtues of activation.

The most intriguing study of activation was that of Borchgrevink et al.[9] They enrolled 201 patients with acute neck pain within 14 days after whiplash. All patients received instructions for self-training of the neck beginning on the first day of treatment, and a 5-day prescription for non-steroidal anti-inflammatory agents. Thereafter patients were randomized to receive the index treatment or a control treatment that consisted of 14-days' sick-leave, and a collar and analgesics for that period. At 6 weeks and at 6 months after treatment, there were no consistent or systematic differences in outcome between the two groups. However, those patients who had the index therapy had slightly lower pain scores at 6 months, and a greater proportion (48% vs 34%) were no longer bothered by neck pain. Reciprocally, slightly fewer (11% vs 15%) still suffered severe symptoms. The index therapy consisted of no more than instructions to act as usual.

These results show that instruction to act as usual is no less effective than a classical regimen of rest, analgesia, and a collar, and is marginally more effective. It is also no less effective than most other passive interventions (see below).

Like reassurance, activation is not a simple, nor a dismissive, intervention. It is not tantamount to telling the patient to ignore the complaint and get on with life. It requires engaging patients, understanding their required and desired activities, encouraging them to resume those activities, and helping them do so. It requires concerted effort on the part of the practitioner, not only to be convincing and credible but also to resist resorting to passive interventions. Furthermore, reassurance cannot be achieved in a short consultation. It takes time to gain the patient's confidence, achieve understanding, and have them be convinced.

REFERENCES

1. Australian Acute Musculoskeletal Pain Guidelines Group. Evidence-Based Management of Acute Musculoskeletal Pain. Australian Academic Press, Brisbane, 2003. (Online. Available at http://www.nhmrc.gov.au/publications/synopses/cp94syn.htm)
2. Spitzer WO, Skovron ML, Salmi LR et al. Scientific monograph of the Quebec Task Force on whiplash-associated disorders: redefining "whiplash" and its management. Spine 1995; 20(Suppl. 8): 1–73.
3. Peeters GGM, Verhagen AP, de Bie RA, Oostendorp RAB. The efficacy of conservative treatment in patients with whiplash injury: a systematic review of clinical trials. Spine 2001; 26: E64–E73.
4. Verhagen AP, Peeters GGM, de Bie RA, Oostendorp RAB. Conservative treatment for whiplash. In: The Cochrane Library; Issue 2. Update Software, Oxford, 2002.
5. Bogduk N, McGuirk B. The evidence. In: Bogduk N, McGuirk B. Medical Management of Acute and Chronic Low Back Pain: An Evidence-Based Approach. Elsevier, Amsterdam, 2002: 83–112.
6. McKinney LA, Dornan JO, Ryan M. The role of physiotherapy in the management of acute neck sprains following road-traffic accidents. Arch Emergency Med 1989; 6: 27–33.
7. McKinney LA. Early mobilisation and outcomes in acute sprains of the neck. Brit Med J 1989; 299: 1006–1008.
8. Rosenfeld M, Gunnarsson R, Borenstein P. Early intervention in whiplash-associated disorders: a comparison of two treatment protocols. Spine 2000; 25: 1782–1787.
9. Borchgrevink GE, Kaasa A, McDonagh D, Stiles TC, Haraldseth O, Lereim I. Acute treatment of whiplash neck sprain injuries: a randomised trial of treatment during the first 14 days after a car accident. Spine 1998; 23: 25–31.

EXERCISES

For the treatment of acute neck pain, two lines of evidence obtain for exercises. There have been studies of exercises coupled only with activation, and studies of exercises as part of a multimodal intervention.

One study compared verbal advice reinforced by written instructions on posture and simple home exercises with rest and analgesia and with active physiotherapy which included manual therapy.[1] It found that simple home exercises were more effective than rest and analgesia, and no less effective than active physiotherapy, at 2 months after treatment. In both the physiotherapy group and the exercise group, pain scores were reduced from 5 to 2, whereas in the rest group they fell only from 5.6 to 3 (Table 10.1).

A supplementary report[2] revealed that at 2 years after treatment, significantly more of those patients treated with advice and home exercises (77%) were pain-free, compared to those treated with rest (54%) or physiotherapy (56%). There was a high drop-out rate (27%) in this follow-up study which theoretically might prejudice the conclusions. However, even if the available data are subjected to worst-case analysis, to adjust for the drop-out, the results still favor home exercises.

Table 10.1 Outcomes of patients with acute neck pain treated in three different ways, as reported by McKinney et al[1] and McKinney[2].

Outcome measure	Rest N = 33	Treatment group Tailored physiotherapy N = 71	Home exercises N = 66
Pain score (0–10)			
—inception	5.6	5.3	5.3
—2 months	3.0	1.9	1.8
Free of pain at 2 years	54%	56%	77%

This conclusion has been reinforced in a more recent study,[3] in which one group of patients was instructed to perform gentle, active, small range and small amplitude rotational movements. The exercises were to be performed 10 times every waking hour. A comparison group was provided with a leaflet providing information about injury mechanisms, advice on suitable activities, and instructions on postural correction, supplemented with a collar. At 6 months after treatment the exercise group showed an average 80% reduction in pain; 38% of the patients were pain-free, and 52% had only low levels of pain. The comparison group showed no reduction in pain; only 17% were pain-free and 30% had low levels of pain. This study also found that outcomes were better if patients were treated within 96 hours after onset of neck pain.

In this study, the odds ratio for achieving complete relief of pain was 2.9 with 95% confidence intervals of 1.1–7.8. For achieving an outcome of little or no pain, the odds ratio was 10.4 (95% CI: 2.4–41.3), which indicates a strong effect. A long-term follow-up of this study reported that the results and differences were sustained over 12 months.[4]

Other studies (see below) have included exercises coupled with manual therapy, as part of a multimodal intervention. It is difficult to distinguish the extent to which the efficacy of the intervention was attributable to the manual therapy, the combination, or to exercises alone. Analysis of the studies suggests that the latter applies.

REFERENCES

1. McKinney LA, Dornan JO, Ryan M. The role of physiotherapy in the management of acute neck sprains following road-traffic accidents. Arch Emergency Med 1989; 6: 27–33.

2. McKinney LA. Early mobilisation and outcomes in acute sprains of the neck. Brit Med J 1989; 299: 1006–1008.

3. Rosenfeld M, Gunnarsson R, Borenstein P. Early intervention in whiplash-associated disorders: a comparison of two treatment protocols. Spine 2000; 25: 1782–1787.

4. Rosenfeld M, Seferiadis A, Carlsson J, Gunnarsson R. Active intervention in patients with whiplash-associated disorders improves long-term prognosis: a randomized controlled trial. Spine 2003; 28: 2491–2498.

MULTIMODAL THERAPY

There have been several studies in which manual therapy, in the form of passive cervical mobilization, has been combined with exercises and other interventions to various extents. To different degrees they provide evidence of the efficacy of these combined regimens.

The oldest study[1] randomly allocated patients to one of two treatment regimens. The index treatment consisted of mobilization using the Maitland technique, together with daily application of heat, and a regimen of daily exercises. The comparison treatment consisted of a soft collar and advice to rest for 2 weeks. Both groups were allowed analgesics. Outcomes were reported in terms of mean pain scores at 4 weeks and 8 weeks after treatment. No subsequent follow-up was provided.

In the index group, mean pain scores fell from 5.7 at inception to 1.7 at 8 weeks. For the control group the corresponding figures were 6.4 and 3.9. The difference amounts to an effect-size of 0.7, which is moderately large. What the study did not report is what proportion of patients were fully relieved of their pain, and what proportion experienced either no relief or a deterioration. The statistics reported suggest that there must have been patients in each of these categories. There was considerable variance in the outcomes of the index treatment group. The standard deviation of the 1.7 score at 8 weeks was 2.3. This implies that 65% of patients had scores across the range from 0.6 to 4.0 with some 17% of patients having even higher scores.

A second study[2] compared the outcomes of patients treated simply with rest and analgesia with those of patients treated with a program of physiotherapy tailored to suit individual patient needs; this included thermal modalities, shortwave diathermy, hydrotherapy, Maitland mobilization, and McKenzie exercises. At 2 months follow-up, the outcomes favored tailored physiotherapy over rest and analgesia (Table 10.1).

A third study[3] evaluated treatment using a collar against the efficacy of a combined regimen of cervical passive mobilization, traction, strengthening exercises, and proprioceptive exercises. It found that a greater proportion of those who received multimodal therapy had recovered at 2 weeks. However, by 12 weeks there were no significant differences between the two treatment groups. A statistical analysis[4] calculated a treatment advantage of only 5.5% in favor of multimodal therapy.

A small study[5] compared the effectiveness of a regimen of cervical mobilization, postural exercises, and advice with that of rest in a collar for 3 weeks. At 3 weeks, significantly fewer patients treated with active therapy still had neck pain than those treated with a collar.

These outcomes were echoed in a repetition of the same study in another setting.[6] At 6 weeks, significantly fewer patients treated with exercise and mobilization still had neck pain than did those treated with a collar.

A rigorous study[7] assessed a multimodal package consisting of relaxation training based on diaphragmatic breathing, postural re-education, psychological support, proprioceptive exercise, and cervical passive mobilization. The comparison treatment was application of transcutaneous electrical nerve stimulation (TENS), pulsed electromagnetic therapy, ultrasound and calcic iontophoresis. At 1 and 6 months after treatment, the multimodal group exhibited significantly lower pain scores. Although the authors did not provide any data on the variance of their outcomes, a systematic review[4] derived an effect-size of 0.79 (95% CI: 1.32, 0.26). At 6 months, 12 out of 30 patients in the multimodal group reported marked improvement but only seven were fully recovered. In the control group, the corresponding figures were two and one, respectively, out of 30 patients.

A conspicuous feature of this study was the poor outcome in the control group. Those patients exhibited virtually no improvement, which does not reflect the responses of control groups in all other studies of acute neck pain. Even patients treated with rest and analgesia typically show modest improvements. This dissonance amplifies the attributable effect of multimodal treatment in this study. A further limitation is that the results cannot be extended to all patients with acute neck pain. The study explicitly excluded patients with 'symptom exaggeration with the intention of enhancing financial rewards.'

The most recent study was reported in two sources: a published paper that reported results at 7 weeks,[8] and a thesis that reported longer term outcomes of the same study.[9] It studied 60 patients treated with multimodal therapy, 59 patients treated with physical therapy, and 64 patients who received usual care from their general practitioner. Some 30% of the patients treated by manual therapy or physical therapy had chronic neck pain, as did 20% of those treated by their general practitioner. About 50% of patients in each group had acute neck pain of less than 6 weeks' duration. The remainder had subacute neck pain. The majority of patients, therefore, qualified as having acute neck pain.

Multimodal therapy involved a variety of techniques directed at mobilizing and stabilizing the cervical spine. The physical therapy consisted of exercises, manual traction, massage, and application of heat. GP care consisted of advice on prognosis and home exercises, encouragement to await spontaneous recovery, and prescription of analgesics.

The published paper[8] reported that the success rate was significantly greater among those patients who were treated with multimodal therapy. "Success rate" was a subjective measure, defined as the proportion of patients who felt that they had either "completely recovered" or were "much improved." However, the results did not identify the proportion of patients who fell into each of these two categories. Instead a single figure was reported that embraced both categories of outcome, and which was deemed to indicate successful outcome. In those terms, 68% of the patients treated with manual therapy had recovered at 7 weeks, compared with 51% of patients treated by physical therapy and 36% of patients under GP care.

Differences in outcomes in more objective measures were less consistent between groups and less in magnitude. At 7 weeks, patients treated by manual therapy exhibited a 56% reduction in pain, on average, compared with 39% for patients treated by physical therapy and 30% for patients under GP care.[8] The reduction in pain in the manual therapy group was significantly greater than in the GP group, but not significantly greater than in the physical therapy group. Reductions in disability, however, amounted to only about 30%, and were not significantly different between groups.[8] Improvements in quality of life measures were 22% for manual therapy, 12% for physical therapy, and 10% for GP care.

The effect-sizes for relief of pain by manual therapy were small (0.3) when compared with physical therapy, but medium (0.7) when compared with GP care. Similarly, the effect-size for reduction of disability by manual therapy was small (0.3) compared with physical therapy, and medium (0.6) when compared with GP care. For improvement in quality of life, the effect-size for manual therapy was barely greater than that of physical therapy (0.01) and was medium (0.5) when compared with GP care.

An editorial that accompanied the paper raised concerns about the subjective nature of "perceived recovery" as an outcome measure, and questioned if manual therapy appeared more successful because of the intensity of the patient–therapist interactions associated with manual therapy.[10] This could be an important factor in light of the fact that whereas patients treated by manual therapy averaged six visits, those under GP care averaged only two visits.[8]

The thesis[9] revealed that with the passage of time, the outcomes in the manual therapy group remained stable while those in the physical therapy and GP groups improved. At 13 weeks, a significantly greater proportion of patients (72%) in the manual therapy than in the GP group (42%) felt that they had recovered, but in neither of these groups was the proportion significantly different from that in the physical therapy group (59%). Patients in the manual therapy group were slightly less disabled than those in the GP group, but were not less disabled than those in physical therapy group. However, pain scores were not significantly different between any of the groups. By 52 weeks, no differences in any outcome measures persisted between groups.

The results of this study show that in terms of objective outcome measures, manual therapy is barely more effective than physical therapy, and is superior to GP care only in the short term. Differences attenuate by 13 weeks, and are absent at 1 year. A greater proportion of patients treated by manual therapy, however, feel recovered at 7 weeks and 13 weeks.

ANALYSIS

The literature on multimodal therapy shows various outcomes. Some regimens are more effective than control treatments in the short term[1,3,5] but in the longer term, outcomes attenuate[3] or have not been studied.[1,5] When long-term outcomes have been reported, the results favor multimodal therapy.[7,8]

What is not immediately evident from the studies is the extent to which individual components of multimodal packages contribute to the observed success. However, two studies do provide data that permit an analysis.

McKinney et al.[2] found tailored physiotherapy to be more effective than rest and analgesia. Their study, however, included a third arm, of patients treated with home exercises. At 2-month follow-up, home exercises were no less effective than tailored physiotherapy. Furthermore, a 2-year follow-up revealed that of patients treated with home exercises, 77% were pain-free, whereas only 56% and 54% of patients in the two other groups were pain-free.[11] These differences are significant statistically. The odds ratio for complete recovery, comparing tailored physiotherapy with rest, is only 1.3, with 95% confidence intervals of 0.8–2.0. This range of values precludes inferring any difference in outcome between the two treatments. However, the odds ratio for home exercises compared with physiotherapy was 2.7 (95% CI: 1.8–3.9). Compared with rest it was 2.9 (95% CI: 1.7–4.9). In both instances, these values indicate a moderate effect in favor of home exercises.

Exercises were a component of the tailored physiotherapy, yet exercises alone were no less effective.

This lack of contrast suggests that exercises are the key component of multimodal therapy, and that other components lack an attributable effect. The second study reinforces this interpretation.

The multimodal therapy of Hoving et al.[8] consisted of passive mobilization and stabilizing exercises. In the short term, it was demonstrably more effective than GP care. The physiotherapy arm of this study used exercises. Multimodal therapy was not consistently and significantly more effective than physiotherapy. This lack of difference again implies that exercises were the key ingredient of the multimodal therapy. The competing interpretation is that none of the overt interventions was the key component but the success was due to the attention provided to the patients, which was substantially greater in both the multimodal group and the physiotherapy group than in the GP group.

Thus, although the data support multimodal therapy as an intervention, it may be that the evidence reinforces the efficacy of exercises for acute neck pain, rather than a particular efficacy of multimodal therapy. Moreover, it is intriguing that the other cardinal component of multimodal therapy is passive cervical mobilization (i.e. manual therapy), yet it has been shown that when used alone cervical mobilization is not effective.[4] Under those circumstances, it becomes difficult to avoid attributing the observed effect of multimodal therapy to anything other than the exercise component.

REFERENCES

1. Mealy K, Brennan H, Fenelon GCC. Early mobilisation of acute whiplash injuries. Brit Med J 1986; 292: 656–657.
2. McKinney LA, Dornan JO, Ryan M. The role of physiotherapy in the management of acute neck sprains following road-traffic accidents. Arch Emergency Med 1989; 6: 27–33.
3. Giebel GD, Edelmann M, Huser R. Die Distorsion der Halswirbelsaule: fruhfunktionelle vs ruhigstellende Behandlung. Zentralblatt fur Chirurgie 1997; 51: 377–384.
4. Gross AR, Kay T, Hondras M, Goldsmith C, Haines T, Peloso P, Kennedy C, Hoving J. Manual therapy for mechanical neck disorders: a systematic review. Man Ther 2002; 7: 131–149.
5. Bonk AD, Ferrari R, Giebel GD, Edelmann M, Huser R. Prospective randomized controlled study of activity vs collar and the natural history of whiplash injury in Germany. J Musculoskeletal Pain 2000; 8: 123–132.
6. Schnabel M, Ferrari R, Vassiliou T, Kaluza G. Randomised, controlled outcome study of active mobilisation compared with collar therapy for whiplash injury. Emerg Med 2004; 21: 306–310.
7. Provinciali L, Baroni M, Illuminati L, Ceravolo MG. Multi-modal treatment to prevent the late whiplash syndrome. Scand J Rehab Med 1996; 28: 105–111.
8. Hoving JL, Koes BW, de Vet CW et al. Manual therapy, physical therapy, or continued care by a general practitioner for patients with neck pain. Ann Int Med 2002; 136: 713–722.

9. Hoving JL. Neck Pain in Primary Care. PhD Thesis, Vrie Universitet, Amsterdam, 2001.
10. Posner J, Glew C. Editorial. Neck pain. Ann Int Med 2002; 136: 758–759.
11. McKinney LA. Early mobilisation and outcomes in acute sprains of the neck. Brit Med J 1989; 299: 1006–1008.

COMPARISON

The relative efficacy of various interventions for acute neck pain can be judged by comparing their outcomes at a selected time after treatment. An appetite outcome measure is the proportion of patients completely relieved of their pain. Not only is this an unambiguous outcome it is also the outcome most desired by patients.

Too few studies have reported outcomes in these terms to allow a comparison of short-term results, but enough studies have reported this outcome at 6 months after treatment to allow a comparison between several interventions (Figure 10.1).

It is evident that several interventions have similar outcomes. They each achieve complete relief of pain in between 40% and 60% of patients at 6 months. They include not only multimodal therapy and exercise therapy, but also conventional care by a general practitioner. Conspicuously, the outcomes of these interventions are not statistically different from those obtained with no passive interventions but only instructions to resume normal activities.[1]

The results obtained in one study of multimodal therapy[3] appear to be statistically greater, but in that study the proportion of patients considered to have a successful outcome included not only those completely recovered (as in the other studies) but also those "much improved." That inclusion is likely to have inflated the proportion. Therefore, the true proportion of patients fully recovered is unlikely to be different from those in the other studies.

This lack of difference between studies in long-term outcome indicates that greater efficacy is not grounds for selecting one intervention over another. By 6 months, all interventions are equal in effect. The option arises, therefore, to select an intervention on other grounds such as simplicity, availability, or pragmatism.

Attractive to some practitioners, and perhaps to insurers, may be the simplicity of assisting patients to resume normal activities, without resorting to any passive interventions. Others might prefer the pragmatism of referring the patient to the care of someone else who might implement exercises or multimodal therapy. If multimodal therapy is not available, exercises are an equivalent substitute; but so too is conventional care.

REFERENCES

1. Borchgrevink GE, Kaasa A, McDonagh D, Stiles TC, Haraldseth O, Lereim I. Acute treatment of whiplash neck sprain injuries: a randomised trial of treatment during the first 14 days after a car accident. Spine 1998; 23: 25–31.
2. Rosenfeld M, Gunnarsson R, Borenstein P. Early intervention in whiplash-associated disorders: a comparison of two treatment protocols. Spine 2000; 25: 1782–1787.
3. Hoving JL. Neck Pain in Primary Care. PhD Thesis, Vrie Universitet, Amsterdam, 2001.
4. Provinciali L, Baroni M, Illuminati L, Ceravolo MG. Multi-modal treatment to prevent the late whiplash syndrome. Scand J Rehab Med 1996; 28: 105–111.

RESERVATIONS

Previous systematic reviews endorsed activation and exercise as the preferred interventions for neck pain.[1,2] The most recent Cochrane review still supports this preference but with less confidence.[3] The basis for this change is a more critical analysis of the literature. For example, in the revision, the studies of McKinney[4,5] are rated as low quality, for a variety of technical reasons. Consequently, the strength of the support for exercises as an intervention falls. As well, the authors of the review carefully analyzed the data presented in the publications and found that often those data did not fully confirm the positive conclusions of the study.[3] The revised conclusions of the review were:

"There seems to be a trend that active interventions are probably more effective than passive intervention, but no clear conclusion can be drawn."

"There is limited evidence that either active or passive treatment is more effective than no treatment."

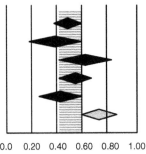

Resume activities [1]
Exercises, self [2]
Exercises, physiotherapy [3]
GP care [3]
Multimodal therapy [4]
Multimodal therapy [3]

0.0   0.20   0.40   0.60   0.80   1.00
Proportion

Figure 10.1 The outcomes at 6 months of various interventions for acute neck pain. The black diamonds indicate the proportion of patients, and 95% confidence limits, who achieved complete relief of pain. The shaded diamond reflects the proportion of patients who either achieved complete relief or were much improved. The shaded zone is the range of proportions over which the confidence limits of the several outcomes overlap.

These conclusions reflect the parlous state of evidence on the treatment of acute neck pain. However, they stem from a demanding and rigorous assessment of the quality of the literature. If studies such as that of McKinney[4,5] are to be ignored, for lack of quality, we are faced with the prospect of having no evidence on which to base the management of acute neck pain.

REFERENCES

1. Peeters GGM, Verhagen AP, de Bie RA, Oostendorp RAB. The efficacy of conservative treatment in patients with whiplash injury: a systematic review of clinical trials. Spine 2001; 26: E64–E73.
2. Verhagen AP, Peeters GGM, de Bie RA, Oostendorp RAB. Conservative treatment for whiplash. In: The Cochrane Library; Issue 2. Update Software, Oxford, 2002.
3. Verhagen AP, Peeters GGM, de Bie RA, Bierma-Zeinstra SMA. Conservative treatment for whiplash. The Cochrane Database of Systematic Reviews, 2004, Issue 1. Art. No. CD003338.pub2. DOI: 10.1002/14651858.CD003338.pub2.
4. McKinney LA, Dornan JO, Ryan M. The role of physiotherapy in the management of acute neck sprains following road-traffic accidents. Arch Emergency Med 1989; 6: 27–33.
5. McKinney LA. Early mobilisation and outcomes in acute sprains of the neck. Brit Med J 1989; 299: 1006–1008.

DRUG THERAPY

ANALGESICS AND NSAIDS

Conspicuously, there have been no studies to show that analgesics or non-steroidal anti-inflammatory drugs (NSAIDs) are effective explicitly for acute neck pain.[1] There are not even inferential data from studies in which these drugs have been used as control treatments. A systematic review[2] identified two studies where the latter could have been the case. One reported that a topical anti-inflammatory agent combined with transcutaneous electrical nerve stimulation (TENS) was superior to TENS alone,[3] but the study was regarded as low quality by the reviewers, who also could not calculate the effect size.[2] The other involved a subgroup of patients with neck pain who were treated either with analgesics, NSAIDs, and education or with placebo consisting of detuned ultrasound.[4] It found no difference in outcome, but the sample sizes were too small to state conclusively that no difference exists.[2]

Nor is there any consolation to be obtained by extrapolating from the literature on low back pain. For acute low back pain, the literature provides little support for analgesics, and shows that NSAIDs are not more effective than placebo for the relief of pain.[5] When used for acute spinal pain, NSAIDs do appear to work, but nearly all of the observed effect can be attributed to the natural resolution of the pain.

Physicians may be drawn to prescribing analgesics or NSAIDs for acute neck pain, as something that they might and can do. However, in that event they should realize that they are prescribing agents that may have no effect greater than placebo, and that prescribing them may be no more than symbolic. Instead of routinely prescribing analgesics, physicians might care to implement other measures that may be safer, and more consonant with the available evidence (see Chapter 9).

MUSCLE RELAXANTS

Diazepam and phenobarbital have been tested, and found to have no greater effect than placebo for the treatment of acute neck pain.[6]

OPIOIDS

Idiopathic acute neck pain is rarely severe enough to invite the use of opioids. If drawn to prescribe opioids, physicians should consider carefully why they are doing so, and whether or not they are missing something. Pain severe enough to require opioids should be urgently investigated for its cause.

KEY POINTS

- There is no direct evidence that analgesics or NSAIDs are effective for acute neck pain.

- For spinal pain in general, these agents are no more effective than the natural history of the condition.

- Muscle relaxants are not effective for acute neck pain.

- Unless there is a serious cause for the pain, which requires urgent diagnosis and treatment in its own right, opioids are not indicated for acute neck pain.

REFERENCES

1. Harms-Ringdahl K, Nachemson A. Acute and subacute neck pain: nonsurgical treatment. In: Nachemson A, Jonsson E (eds). Neck and Back Pain: The Scientific Evidence of Causes, Diagnosis, and Treatment. Lippincott Williams and Wilkins, Philadelphia, 2000: 327–338.
2. Aker PD, Gross AR, Goldsmith CH, Peloso P. Conservative management of mechanical neck pain: systematic overview and meta-analysis. Brit Med J 1996; 313: 1291–1296.
3. Coletta R, Maggiolo F, di Tizio S. Etofenamate and transcutaneous electrical nerve stimulation treatment of painful spinal syndromes. Int Clin Pharmacol Res 1988; 8: 295–298.

4. Koes BW, Bouter LM, van Mameren H et al. The effectiveness of manual therapy, physiotherapy, and treatment by the general practitioner for nonspecific back and neck complaints: a randomized clinical trial. Spine 1992; 17: 28–35.
5. Bogduk N. Pharmacological alternatives for the alleviation of back pain. Expert Opin Phamacother 2004; 5: 2091–2098.
6. Basmajian JV. Reflex cervical muscle spasm: treatment by diazepam, phenobarbital or placebo. Arch Phys Med Rehabil 1983; 64: 121–124.

SPRAY AND STRETCH

One method advocated for the treatment of myofascial pain is to spray the affected area with a vapocoolant to induce analgesia, and subsequently to stretch the underlying muscle. This treatment has been studied, but reported only in abstract form.[1] Nevertheless, the study was rated as methodologically strong by one systematic review.[2] The results showed no effect greater than that of placebo.[1]

The review accepted this study as providing evidence that spray and stretch was not effective for neck pain.[2] Another review[3] noted the negative result but commented that because of the small size of this study, the result should be interpreted with caution.

It is unfortunate that this study has not appeared in the form of a full paper, and that no other studies of this commonly used treatment have been conducted. What is plain, however, is that the only available evidence does not support this form of treatment.

KEY POINT

- Spray and stretch therapy is no more effective than placebo therapy

REFERENCES

1. Snow CJ, Aves Wood R, Dowhopouuk H et al. Randomized controlled clinical trail of spray and stretch for relief of back and neck myofascial pain. (Abstract). Physiotherapy Canada 1992; 44: 2 S8.
2. Aker PD, Gross AR, Goldsmith CH, Peloso P. Conservative management of mechanical neck pain: systematic overview and meta-analysis. Brit Med J 1996; 313: 1291–1296.
3. Harms-Ringdahl K, Nachemson A. Acute and subacute neck pain: nonsurgical treatment. In: Nachemson A, Jonsson E (eds). Neck and Back Pain: The Scientific Evidence of Causes, Diagnosis, and Treatment. Lippincott Williams and Wilkins, Philadelphia, 2000: 327–338.

ACUPUNCTURE

There is very little literature on the efficacy of acupuncture for acute neck pain. Two systematic reviews[1,2] identified the same two studies.[3,4] One of these reviews, however, considered both studies to have included chronic patients, and did not consider them to have provided evidence on the treatment of acute neck pain.[2]

Whereas one of the two studies was explicit in having recruited patients with chronic neck pain,[3] the other[4] was ambiguous in its reporting. It did not stipulate the duration of symptoms, but did comment that "duration of symptoms prior to treatment was found to have no relationship to its outcome."[4] Furthermore, patients were recruited who had not received previous treatment apart from simple analgesic agents, which suggests that they were unlikely to have had prolonged symptoms.

That study[4] was rated as poor in methodological quality[1] and did not provide data from which an effect size could be calculated.[1] The study compared the outcomes of electroacupuncture and physiotherapy. The study was not blinded; statistical analysis was not performed; the conclusions were tentative and modest, viz.: "electroacupuncture can bring about earlier symptomatic improvement with increased neck movements, especially in patients with less severe degenerative changes in their cervical spine."

The study reported that patients treated with electroacupuncture, on average reported a greater percentage improvement in their pain, but the distributions of responses were not reported. For this reason, a systematic review was unable to extract an effect size.[1] However, the proportion of patients who obtained complete relief was the same for both treatments.

For lack of blinding in the study, and for lack of detailed statistical results, this study falls short of constituting positive evidence of the efficacy of acupuncture for neck pain. At best, the results suggest that electroacupuncture may be modestly superior to physiotherapy, but the lack of blinding constitutes a fatal flaw for even this modest suggestion.

Applying infra-red heat to acupuncture points or to tender points is one alternative to needle acupuncture. This form of therapy has been tested in a randomized study in which mock transcutaneous electrical nerves stimulation (TENS) was used as the control.[5] The study was not blinded, but even so, the results of infra-red therapy were no better than those of sham therapy.

REFERENCES

1. Aker PD, Gross AR, Goldsmith CH, Peloso P. Conservative management of mechanical neck pain: systematic overview and meta-analysis. Brit Med J 1996; 313: 1291–1296.
2. Harms-Ringdahl K, Nachemson A. Acute and subacute neck pain: nonsurgical treatment. In: Nachemson A, Jonsson E (eds). Neck and Back Pain: The Scientific Evidence of Causes, Diagnosis, and Treatment. Lippincott Williams and Wilkins, Philadelphia, 2000: 327–338.
3. Petrie JP, Langley GB. Acupuncture in the treatment of chronic cervical pain: a pilot study. Clin Exp Rheumatol 1983; 1: 333–335.
4. Loy TT. Treatment of cervical spondylosis: electroacupuncture versus physiotherapy. Med J Aust 1983; 2: 32–34.
5. Lewith GT, Machin D. A randomised trial to evaluate the effect of infra-red stimulation of local trigger points, versus placebo on the pain caused by cervical osteoarthrosis. Acupuncture Electro-Therapeut Res Int J 1981; 6: 277–284.

TENS

The literature on transcutaneous electrical nerve stimulation (TENS) for acute neck pain is limited to one study.[1] This small study was of short duration because all patients resolved within 2 weeks. TENS was no more effective than other interventions, such as collar, rest, education, and analgesics.

REFERENCE

1. Nordemar R, Throner C. Treatment of acute cervical pain: a comparative group study. Pain 1981; 10: 93–101.

TRACTION

Systematic reviews have differed in the literature that they have identified concerning traction for acute neck pain. One study,[1] identified by each of two reviews,[2,3] was not a study of neck pain, as patients were recruited expressly for pain radiating into the upper limb. It is, therefore, a study of cervical radicular pain.

Four studies provide data on the efficacy of traction for neck pain. The most recent[4] was identified by both systematic reviews of this subject.[2,3] An older study[5] was additionally identified by the most recent review,[3] but both reviews did not include still older studies.[6,7]

The first of these studies found no added benefit from intermittent traction and exercise instruction over 2 weeks' rest in a standard or molded collar.[4] The second found no differences in pain severity following treatment with static traction, intermittent traction, manual traction, and no traction, when added to a regimen of instruction, moist heat and a program of exercises.[5] The third assessed the value of adding various forms of traction, or no traction, to drug therapy.[6] It found advantage to be gained from adding traction. The fourth did not report whether it studied patients with acute or chronic neck pain,[6] but it found no difference in outcome between patients treated with: (i) heat, massage and traction, (ii) a felt collar, or (iii) exercises.

REFERENCES

1. Goldie I, Landquist A. Evaluation of the effects of different forms of physiotherapy in cervical pain. Scand J Rehab Med 1970; 2–3: 117–121.
2. Aker PD, Gross AR, Goldsmith CH, Peloso P. Conservative management of mechanical neck pain: systematic overview and meta-analysis. Brit Med J 1996; 313: 1291–1296.
3. Harms-Ringdahl K, Nachemson A. Acute and subacute neck pain: nonsurgical treatment. In: Nachemson A, Jonsson E (eds). Neck and Back Pain: The Scientific Evidence of Causes, Diagnosis, and Treatment. Lippincott Williams and Wilkins, Philadelphia, 2000: 327–338.
4. Pennie BH, Agambar LJ. Whiplash injuries: a trial of early management. J Bone Joint Surg 1990; 72B: 277–279.
5. Zylbergold RS, Piper MC. Cervical spine disorders: a comparison of three types of traction. Spine 1985; 10: 867–871.
6. Caldwell JW, Krusen EM. Effectiveness of cervical traction in treatment of neck problems: evaluation of various methods. Arch Phys Med Rehab 1962; 43: 214–221.
7. Steinberg VL, Mason RM. Cervical spondylosis: pilot therapeutic trial. Ann Phys Med 1959; 5: 37–47.

COLLARS

Collars have been evaluated directly or indirectly in many trials of treatment for acute neck pain. At times they have been part of the index treatment.[1,2,3] At other times they have been used as the control treatment [4,5,6] or as a comparison treatment.[7] In only one study have collars been explicitly tested against rest and analgesics.[8] Uniformly, these studies have revealed no benefit from the wearing of collars.

KEY POINT

- Collars confer no benefit for the relief of acute neck pain.

REFERENCES

1. McKinney LA, Dornan JO, Ryan M. The role of physiotherapy in the management of acute neck sprains following road-traffic accidents. Arch Emergency Med 1989; 6: 27–33.
2. Mealy K, Brennan H, Fenelon GCC. Early mobilisation of acute whiplash injuries. Brit Med J 1986; 292: 656–657.
3. Pennie BH, Agambar LJ. Whiplash injuries: a trial of early management. J Bone Joint Surg 1990; 72B: 277–279.
4. Nordemar R, Throner C. Treatment of acute cervical pain: a comparative group study. Pain 1981; 10: 93–101.
5. Rosenfeld M, Gunnarsson R, Borenstein P. Early intervention in whiplash-associated disorders: a comparison of two treatment protocols. Spine 2000; 25: 1782–1787.
6. Borchgrevink GE, Kaasa A, McDonagh D, Stiles TC, Haraldseth O, Lereim I. Acute treatment of whiplash neck sprain injuries: a randomised trial of treatment during the first 14 days after a car accident. Spine 1998; 23: 25–31.
7. Steinberg VL, Mason RM. Cervical spondylosis: pilot therapeutic trial. Ann Phys Med 1959; 5: 37–47.
8. Gennis P, Miller L, Gallagher EJ, Giglio J, Carter W, Nathanson N. The effect of soft collars on persistent neck pain in patients with whiplash injury. Acad Emerg Med 1996; 3: 568–573.

PULSED ELECTROMAGNETIC THERAPY

Two studies of pulsed electromagnetic therapy have been published by the same investigators, using different samples of patients.[1,2] The results were the same in both.

In the first study,[1] patients undergoing the index treatment wore a collar for 8 hours a day, for two consecutive periods of 3 weeks. The collars were embedded with a device that delivered a pulsed electromagnetic stimulus. The patients used a different device for each of the two 3-week periods. The control patients wore a collar in which a placebo device was embedded for the first 3 weeks, but received an active device for the second 3 weeks. This latter permutation precludes drawing inferences about the effectiveness of the active treatment beyond 3 weeks. At the end of the first 3 weeks, those patients treated with an active device reported significantly greater reduction of pain, but there were no differences at 6 weeks. Nor was any longer-term follow-up reported.

In the second study,[2] patients were required to wear a collar for 12 weeks; half the collars were embedded with an active device, and half with a placebo device. Patients treated with the active device exhibited significantly greater reductions in pain at 2 weeks and 4 weeks, but not at 12 weeks. At 4 weeks, a significantly greater proportion of patients treated with the active device reported feeling "moderately better" and few were worse. At 12 weeks, there were no differences between the treatment groups with respect to the proportions of patients feeling "completely well," "much better," "moderately better," "slightly better," "unchanged," or "worse."

This evidence indicates that pulsed electromagnetic therapy has a modest effect in the short term for making some patients feel "moderately" better. It does not result in a greater proportion of patients being completely relieved; and there is no evidence of any lasting effect. The principal disadvantage of this form of therapy is the necessity for patients to wear a collar for 8 hours a day. This seems to be a major inconvenience in light of the limited benefit that the treatment affords.

These studies have consistently been rated as of good quality by systematic reviews.[3,4,5] The most recent review[6] maintained this rating, but discovered that the device was no longer available. This renders pointless the publications describing the efficacy of this intervention.

KEY POINTS

- Pulsed electromagnetic therapy makes some patients feel moderately better,

- but achieves no greater long-term outcome than wearing an inactive collar,

- yet incurs the inconvenience of wearing a collar for 8 hours a day.

REFERENCES

1. Foley-Nolan D, Barry C, Coughlan RJ, O'Connor P, Roden D. Pulsed high frequency (27MHz) electromagnetic therapy for persistent pain: a double blind, placebo-controlled study of 20 patients. Orthopaedics 1990; 13: 445–451.

2. Foley-Nolan D, Moore K, Codd M, Barry C, O'Connor P, Coughlan RJ. Low energy high frequency pulsed electromagnetic therapy for acute whiplash injuries. Scand J Rehab Med 1992; 24: 51–59.
3. Harms-Ringdahl K, Nachemson A. Acute and subacute neck pain: nonsurgical treatment. In: Nachemson A, Jonsson E (eds). Neck and Back Pain: The Scientific Evidence of Causes, Diagnosis, and Treatment. Lippincott Williams and Wilkins, Philadelphia, 2000: 327–338.
4. Peeters GGM, Verhagen AP, de Bie RA, Oostendorp RAB. The efficacy of conservative treatment in patients with whiplash injury. A systematic review of clinical trials. Spine 2001; 26: E64–E73.
5. Verhagen AP, Peeters GGM, de Bie RA, Oostendorp RAB. Conservative treatment for whiplash. In: The Cochrane Library; Issue 2. Update Software, Oxford, 2002.
6. Verhagen AP, Peeters GGM, de Bie RA, Bierma-Zeinstra SMA. Conservative treatment for whiplash. The Cochrane Database of Systematic Reviews, 2004: 1.

MANUAL THERAPY

Manual therapy has been a prominent, if not major, focus in systematic reviews of treatment for neck pain. However, there have been few studies that have provided compelling evidence. Seemingly, in an effort to maximize the data, reviews have included studies that examined only the immediate effects of manual therapy, with no further follow-up; and have relied on studies that included patients with chronic neck pain and patients with acute neck pain, in various proportions, without stratifying the results.[1] Only four studies have explicitly addressed the treatment of acute neck pain, and one has provided data on a mixed sample, the majority of whom were patients with acute or subacute neck pain.

One study reported the immediate effects of manipulation. It compared rotational manipulation with muscle energy therapy.[2] It showed that 85% of patients treated by manipulation reported an immediate reduction in pain, compared with 65% of patients treated with muscle energy therapy. The differences in mean decrease in pain were reported as significantly different statistically, but this significance disappears if the data are adjusted for pre-treatment differences.[1] Even so, the magnitude of the treatment effect amounted to little more than a 12-point improvement on a 100-point scale.

One study compared the efficacy of manipulation with that of treatment with azapropazone, for acute neck pain.[3] It found that immediately after treatment, a significantly greater proportion of patients treated by manipulation showed improvement in neck pain and in other measures; but these differences were extinguished by 1 week and 3 weeks after treatment. This study, therefore, showed that the benefits of manipulation for neck pain were very short-lived.

Three studies have assessed the efficacy of mobilization, as opposed to manipulation, for neck pain. They constitute the principal body of evidence concerning the efficacy of manual therapy for this condition.

A very small study,[4] with a sample size of 10, found no difference in outcome between patients treated with manual therapy and those treated with TENS, or a collar. No differences emerged because all patients in all treatment groups recovered fully within 1 week.

KEY POINTS

In the short-term:

- manual therapy for acute neck pain is more effective than limited usual care by a general practitioner, but

- manual therapy is not more effective than physical therapy, or a home exercise program.

In the long-term:

- manual therapy affords no significant benefit over other interventions for the reduction of neck pain.

REFERENCES

1. Cassidy JD, Lopes AA, Yong-Hing K. The immediate effect of manipulation versus mobilization on pain and range of motion in the cervical spine: a randomized controlled trial. J Manip Physiol Ther 1992; 15: 570–575.
2. Hurwitz EL, Aker PR, Adams AH, Meeker WC, Shekelle PG. Manipulation and mobilization of the cervical spine: a systematic review of the literature. Spine 1996; 21: 1746–1760.
3. Howe DH, Newcombe RG, Wade MT. Manipulation of the cervical spine: pilot study. J Roy Coll Gen Pract 1983; 33: 574–579.
4. Nordemar R, Throner C. Treatment of acute cervical pain: a comparative group study. Pain 1981; 10: 93–101.

MISCELLANEOUS

Neck school has been shown to confer no benefit greater than that of no treatment.[1] Nor does a program of group *gymnastics* reduce neck pain more than natural history and seasonal fluctuations.[2]

Various forms of *electrotherapy* have been studied. One form was found to be as effective as no treatment.[3] Another was more effective than no treatment 15 minutes after treatment, but not at 6 weeks.[4]

No studies have vindicated the treatment of neck pain by *prolotherapy* or other forms of *injections*.

KEY POINT

- Neck school, gymnastics, electrotherapy, and injections are not effective for acute neck pain.

REFERENCES

1. Kamwendo K, Linton SJ. A controlled study of the effect of neck school in medical secretaries. Scand J Rehab Med 1991; 23: 143–152.

2. Takala EP, Viikari-Juntura E, Tynklynen EM. Does group gymnastics at the workplace help in neck pain? Scand J Rehab Med 1994; 26: 17–20.

3. Fialka V, Preisnger E, Bohler A. Zur physikalischen diagnostik ind physikalischer therapie der distorsio columnae cervicalis. Z Phys Med Baln Med Klim 1989; 18: 390–397.

4. Hendriks O, Horgan A. Ultra-Reiz current as an adjunct to standard physiotherapy treatment of the acute whiplash patient. Physiother Ireland 1996; 17: 3–7.

3 Chronic neck pain

11 Chronic neck pain: overview

Despite the best of care during the acute phase, some 20% of patients will continue to suffer persistent pain (Chapter 4). Perhaps the figure may be as high as 40%. These figures will include some 5% or more with severe symptoms. If this pain persists beyond 3 months, by definition it constitutes chronic neck pain.

There is a view that chronic neck pain after whiplash is not due to an organic lesion. Rather, the interpretation is that these patients have a psychosocial basis for their pain. That basis has not been explicitly elaborated, but the implication is that they are malingering, or exaggerating their pain for financial or other rewards. Neither implication is a medical diagnosis. Each is an accusation. Furthermore, systematic reviews have refuted any scientific basis for either malingering[1] or secondary gain.[2]

A further perplexing issue is that patients with idiopathic neck pain also develop chronic symptoms, yet they have nothing to gain from malingering or from a compensation system. Grounds for invoking a psychosocial basis for this form of chronic neck pain, therefore, become tenuous. The only recourse to avoid an organic explanation is to invoke the concept of psychogenic pain, which is not a recognized psychiatric diagnosis.[3] It is a technical-sounding diagnosis that cannot be distinguished from a euphemism for "I don't know why your neck hurts," but one that discharges any blame from the doctor for not knowing, and places it back on the patient.

Nor does a patient with persistent neck pain satisfy the diagnostic criteria for any recognized psychiatric disorder. While so long as all they have is neck pain, they do not satisfy the criteria for somatization disorder, for those criteria require that the patient must have pain in at least four different sites, as well as two gastrointestinal symptoms, one sexual symptom, and one pseudoneurological symptom, the latter not limited to pain.[3] Nor do they have a conversion disorder or hypochondriasis. The essence of conversion disorder is that the patient has a loss of motor or sensory function, such as paralysis, blindness, or numbness. The notes and diagnostic criteria for this rubric specifically preclude its use if pain is the sole symptom.[3] The diagnostic criteria for hypochondriasis stipulate that the patient has a preoccupation with fears of having a serious disease. Although patients with chronic pain may appear preoccupied with their pain, to the extent of seeking relief, this differs from having a preoccupation with a fear of having pain, or fear of a serious disorder.

Persistent neck pain invites, if not mandates, a consideration and pursuit of its cause. Those intent upon applying a psychosocial diagnosis need to distinguish between simply labeling patients and making a valid diagnosis. For a diagnosis to be valid, criteria must be available and those criteria must be satisfied. Conversely, there must be a means of refuting that diagnosis. Pyschosocial diagnoses fail in the latter respect. They are applied ad hoc as no more than a hypothesis, but with no test by which that hypothesis can be rejected. This renders psychosocial labels a belief, not a diagnosis.

For those wishing to pursue a biomedical diagnosis, some evidence is available as to the possible causes of chronic neck pain and how it might be diagnosed.

The evidence is incomplete and for many patients an explanation is not yet available. That unfortunate circumstance, however, is more a reflection of the lack of research into neck pain, to date, than a reason to blame patients.

REFERENCES

1. Fishbain DA, Cutler R, Rosomoff HL, Rosomoff RS. Chronic pain disability exaggeration/malingering and submaximal effort research. Clin J Pain 1999; 15: 244–274.

2. Fishbain DA, Rosomoff HL, Cutler RB, Rosomoff RS. Secondary gain concept: a review of the scientific evidence. Clin J Pain 1995; 11: 6–21.

3. DSM-IV-TR. Diagnostic and Statistical Manual of Mental Disorders, 4th edn. Text Revision. American Psychiatric Association, Washington DC, 2000.

Chronic neck pain: causes

KEY POINTS

- There are no known causes of chronic neck pain in the absence of trauma.

- If osteoarthrosis of the cervical synovial joints is a cause of pain, it cannot be detected validly by radiography.

- The most likely causes of chronic neck pain after trauma are tears of the anterior anulus and various impaction injuries of the zygapophysial joints or lateral atlanto-axial joints.

- Whiplash may produce lesions in the alar and transverse ligaments.

Despite the prevalence of chronic neck pain, little research has gone into understanding its causes. For idiopathic chronic neck pain there is virtually no information concerning its causes. For chronic neck pain after whiplash there is some indication of what its causes might be.

IDIOPATHIC NECK PAIN

Idiopathic neck pain is defined essentially by the absence of trauma, or any other explanation of why the neck pain has started. In anatomical terms the leading possible sources of pain are the muscles, discs, and joints of the cervical spine. In pathologic terms, there are no known or established conditions that might affect these structures so as to generate persistent pain.

MUSCLES

Although muscle sprains might be an explanation for acute neck pain, they do not provide an explanation for chronic neck pain. The natural history of muscle sprains is to heal rapidly, within days.

Entities such as muscle spasm, chronic muscle ischemia, and trigger points have variously been invoked as mechanisms for chronic pain from muscles, but none has been verified clinically. There is no evidence as to how these conditions might be diagnosed or refuted in clinical practice. There is no evidence as to how commonly they occur.

Disturbances of muscle function have been documented as a feature of patients with neck pain.[1,2,3,4] They include weakness of the neck flexors[1] and greater muscle fatigue;[5] but a more complex picture has emerged. Patients with neck pain exhibit impaired function of deep cervical flexors (longus cervicis and capitis)[6] which results in greater activation of superficial flexors (sternocleidomastoid).[7] Moreover, patients exhibit abnormal patterns of activation of accessory neck muscles, such as the anterior scalenes and trapezius.[8]

These abnormal patterns do not constitute a basis for pain, but they implicate a secondary response to pain. They do not correlate with fear-avoidance[4] and so, cannot be ascribed simply to antalgic reactions. They imply disturbed coordination as unaffected muscles compensate for weakened muscles, or they might reflect a higher order of discoordinated motor activity in the central nervous system as a consequence of persistent pain.

REFERENCES

1. Barton PM, Hayes KC. Neck flexor muscle strength, efficiency, and relaxation times in normal subjects and subjects with unilateral neck pain and headache. Arch Phys Med Rehabil 1996; 77: 680–687.
2. Nederhand MJ, Ijzerman MJ, Hermens HJ, Baten CTM, Zivold G. Cervical muscle dysfunction in the chronic whiplash associated disorder grade II (WAD-II). Spine 2000; 25: 1938–1943.
3. Nederhand MJ, Hermens HJ, Ijzerman MJ, Turk DC, Zivold G. Chronic neck pain disability due to an acute whiplash injury. Pain 2003; 102: 63–71.
4. Sterling M, Jull G, Vicenzino B, Kennardy J, Darnell R. Development of motor system dysfunction following whiplash injury. Pain 2003; 103: 65–73.
5. Falla D, Jull G, Rainoldi A, Merletti R. Neck flexor muscle fatigue is side specific in patients with unilateral neck pain. Eur J Pain 2004; 8: 71–77.
6. Falla DL, Jull GA, Hodges PW. Patients with neck pain demonstrate reduced electromyographic activity of the deep cervical flexor muscles during performance of the craniocervical flexion test. Spine 2004; 29: 2108–2114.
7. Jull G, Kristjansson E, Dall'Alba P. Impairment in the cervical flexors: a comparison of whiplash and insidious onset neck pain patients. Man Ther 2004; 9: 89–94.
8. Falla D, Bilenkij G, Jull G. Patients with chronic neck pain demonstrate altered patterns of muscle activation during performance of a functional upper limb task. Spine 2004; 29: 1436–1440.

INTERVERTEBRAL DISCS

No model has been proposed to explain why, or how, a cervical intervertebral disc might become symptomatic in the absence of trauma. Indeed, it is difficult to conceive of such an explanation. There is no reason why an uninjured disc should become painful. There is no reason why age changes should render a disc painful. There is no immediate link between nociception and a disc drying out or developing osteophytes. Recurrent strain, without injury, has not been demonstrated; nor has it ever been formally postulated as the reason why discs become painful.

SYNOVIAL JOINTS

The most attractive explanation for chronic idiopathic neck pain is osteoarthritis of the synovial joints of the neck: the zygapophysial joints at typical cervical levels, and the atlanto-axial and atlanto-occipital joints at upper cervical levels. The problem with this interpretation is that studies have demonstrated that the radiographic changes of osteoarthritis in the cervical spine do not correlate with pain; they are too often present in totally asymptomatic individuals.[1,2]

A reconciliation, nevertheless, is possible. It has been shown that post-mortem studies reveal a greater incidence of osteoarthritis than do radiographic studies of the same spines,[3] particularly at upper cervical levels. Radiography, therefore, may be failing to detect significant numbers of patients with symptomatic osteoarthritis.

In that event, osteoarthritis might well be a valid cause of neck pain, but radiography is not the means by which to diagnose it. Population studies have not shown any utility of CT or MRI in this regard. The only available means of testing if a cervical synovial joint is the source of pain is to anesthetize it (see Chapter 13).

REFERENCES

1. Heller CA, Stanley P, Lewis-Jones B, Heller RF. Value of X-ray examinations of the cervical spine. Brit Med J 1983; 287: 1276–1278.
2. Fridenberg ZB, Miller WT. Degenerative disc disease of the cervical spine: a comparative study of asymptomatic and symptomatic patients. J Bone Joint Surg 1963; 45A: 1171–1178.
3. Sager P. An assessment of the accuracy of radiologic diagnosis in the cervical spine. In: Hirsch C, Zotterman Y (eds). Cervical Pain. Pergamon, Oxford, 1972: 49–52.

NECK PAIN AFTER INJURY

There is somewhat more evidence on the possible causes of chronic neck pain after whiplash. That evidence applies reasonably well also to neck pain after trauma not involving whiplash *per se*.

MUSCLES

As with idiopathic neck pain, there are no grounds for believing that muscles can be the primary source of chronic neck pain after injury. There are no known lesions that both persist over time and cause pain from muscles.

INTERVERTEBRAL DISCS

The biomechanics data (Chapter 17) indicate that extension injuries of the cervical spine can injure the anterior anulus fibrosus (Figure 12.1). The lesion is a tear of the anterior anulus, or an avulsion of the anulus from the vertebral body. It is reasonable to infer that such a lesion would be painful, on the grounds that similar ligament tears elsewhere in the body are accepted as causes of pain. Such lesions of the cervical discs have been demonstrated in post-mortem studies of victims of lethal motor vehicle accidents (Chapter 17).

SYNOVIAL JOINTS

The biomechanics data also indicate that extension injuries of the cervical spine can injure the zygapophysial joints of the neck (Chapter 17). The lesions range from contusions of the intra-articular meniscoids with intra-articular hemorrhage, to subchondral and greater articular fractures (Figure 12.1). Such lesions have been demonstrated both in the cervical zygapophysial joints and in the lateral atlanto-axial joints (Chapter 17). Each of the lesions is a feasible cause of pain, for analogous lesions in joints of the appendicular skeleton are accepted as causes of pain.

ALAR AND TRANSVERSE LIGAMENTS

It is known from the orthopedic literature that the suboccipital ligaments can be ruptured during severe trauma to the head and neck. Affected patients typically present with instability of the atlas, or with features of spinal cord injury.[1,2] Such injuries, however, would not be the basis of uncomplicated neck pain after trauma, i.e. in the absence of instability or neurological signs.

For lesser lesions of the suboccipital ligaments, there is no evidence from biomechanics studies that these ligaments might be injured in whiplash; but this may be because studies have not focused on the suboccipital level. Furthermore, post-mortem studies have not distinguished minor lesions of the suboccipital ligaments from more lethal injuries in this region.[3,4,5,6]

The radiology literature, however, provides preliminary evidence that alar and transverse ligaments *might* be injured in whiplash. A series of MRI studies looked for injuries to these ligaments. They distinguished grade 1, 2, and 3 lesions, according to whether a high-intensity signal was evident across one, two, or three thirds of the cross-sectional area of the ligament. They found lesions to be significantly more common in subjects with a history of whiplash than in asymptomatic individuals (Table 12.1).

These data constitute prima facie evidence that lesions of the suboccipital ligaments might be a feature of whiplash. In that regard, grade 2 and grade 3 lesions of the alar ligaments are the most common, and were not found in asymptomatic controls (Table 12.1). Lesions of the transverse ligament were less common in patients with a history of whiplash, but occurred also in asymptomatic subjects.

It is not evident if these lesions are symptomatic or not, for the studies did not report what symptoms the patients had. If these lesions are symptomatic, their location at the C1 level renders them a potential source of cervicogenic headache, rather than neck pain. If not symptomatic, these lesions may nonetheless constitute a coincidental sign of injury.

Table 12.1 The prevalence of different grades of lesions of the alar and transverse ligaments in patients with whiplash and in control asymptomatic subjects. Based on Krakenes et al.[7,8]

		Whiplash	Control
Alar ligament[7]	Lesions		
	Grade 1	29	4
	Grade 2	27	0
	Grade 3	18	0
	Normal	18	26
Transverse ligament[8]	Lesions		
	Grade 1	10	3
	Grade 2	16	3
	Grade 3	5	0
	Normal	61	24

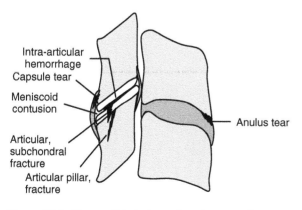

Intra-articular hemorrhage
Capsule tear
Meniscoid contusion
Articular, subchondral fracture
Articular pillar, fracture
Anulus tear

Figure 12.1 The possible lesions of post-traumatic neck pain.

Replication studies are required to establish if these lesions are valid. Those studies should determine if the lesions can be detected by others; if they occur in other samples of patients with whiplash; and if they correlate with symptoms.

REFERENCES

1. Levine AM, Edwards CC. Traumatic lesions of the occipitoatlantoaxial complex. Clin Orthop 1989; 239: 53–56.
2. An H. Cervical spine trauma. Spine 1998; 23: 2713–2729.
3. Jónsson H, Bring G, Rauschning W, Sahlstedt B. Hidden cervical spine injuries in traffic accident victims with skull fractures. J Spinal Disorders 1991; 4: 251–263.
4. Taylor JR, Twomey LT. Acute injuries to cervical joints: an autopsy study of neck sprain. Spine 1993; 9: 1115–1122.
5. Taylor JR, Taylor MM. Cervical spinal injuries: an autopsy study of 109 blunt injuries. J Musculoskelet Pain 1996; 4: 61–79.
6. Uhrenholdt L, Grunnet-Nilsson N, Hartvigsen K. Cervical spine lesions after road traffic accidents: a systematic review. Spine 2002; 27: 1934–1941.
7. Krakenes J, Kaale BR, Moen G, Nordli H, Gilhus NE, Rorvik J. MRI assessment of the alar ligaments in the late stage of whiplash injury: a study of structural abnormalities and observer agreement. Neuroradiology 2002; 44: 617–624.
8. Krakenes J, Kaale BR, Moen G, Nordli H, Rorvik J, Gilhus NE. MR analysis of the transverse ligament in the late stage of whiplash injury. Acta Radiol 2003; 44: 637–644.

13

Chronic neck pain: investigations

KEY POINTS

- Conventional medical imaging does not reveal causes of chronic neck pain in most patients.

- Radiographs and CT scans are not indicated for chronic neck pain. They are not able to reveal lesions that are the basis for chronic neck pain.

- MRI does not reveal common lesions.

- Nevertheless, MRI is the best screening tool for possibly occult lesions.

- For its diagnosis, pain requires a physiological test.

- Pain stemming from cervical intervertebral discs can be diagnosed by cervical discography;

but

- the prevalence of cervical discogenic pain has not been determined.

- pain stemming from cervical zygapophysial joints can be diagnosed by controlled, diagnostic blocks of the medial branches that innervate them.

- cervical zygapophysial joint pain is the single most common basis for chronic neck pain.

- it accounts for over 50% of patients with chronic neck pain after whiplash.

The objective of investigations is to pinpoint the source of pain and its cause. For chronic neck pain, medical imaging has a limited role. Other investigations are more appropriate.

MEDICAL IMAGING

The utility of medical imaging in the pursuit of pain is limited by what the test can show and the prevalence of the lesions that can be demonstrated. Few of the lesions that might account for chronic neck pain (Chapter 12) can be demonstrated by conventional medical imaging.

PLAIN RADIOGRAPHY

Plain radiography shows the state of bones and joints, and may demonstrate the late stages of tumors or infections. Tumors and infections, however, are rare causes of neck pain and are better demonstrated by other techniques. Major fractures are unlikely to account for chronic neck pain, for they are likely to have been detected during the acute phase. If major fractures escaped detection according to the Canadian C-spine rule (Chapter 7), because they did not impede neck movements during the acute phase, their relevance to chronic pain becomes questionable. They may be no more than an incidental finding.

Plain radiography lacks sensitivity for small fractures of the cervical spine, such as those affecting the zygapophysial joints, articular pillars, and laminae. Nevertheless, it might detect such fractures or show suspicious signs suggestive of such fractures. CT provides better resolution of these small fractures.

CT SCANNING

Several studies have directed attention to small fractures of the articular pillars or facets of the cervical zygapophysial joints.[1-5] Some 87% of these are not detected by plain radiography, but they can be detected by CT. Some studies suggest that they account for up to 20% of fractures of the cervical spine.[2,3,4]

These data, however, do not justify a search for small fractures in all patients with chronic neck pain. In the first instance, their low prevalence means that investigations are unlikely to be positive. Secondly, there are no indications for where to look. If the fracture could be anywhere, the entire cervical spine would have to be subjected to high-resolution scanning, which involves considerable radiation exposure to the patient. Thirdly, detecting small fractures may be of no more than academic interest, for there is no specific management that could be instituted, or needs to be instituted. Fourthly, finding such a fracture does not necessarily implicate it as the source of pain. There is no evidence, to date, that these fractures are symptomatic, or that they are any more than incidental findings.

For these reasons, CT to look for small fractures has no place in the routine management of patients with chronic neck pain. It is essentially a research tool, able to provide good resolution of these lesions, whose clinical significance has not been established.

REFERENCES

1. Lee C, Woodring JH. Sagittally oriented fractures of the lateral masses of the cervical vertebrae. J Trauma 1991; 31: 1638–1643.
2. Clark CR, Igram CM, El-Khoury GY, Ehara S. Radiographic evaluation of cervical spine injuries. Spine 1988; 13: 742–747.
3. Woodring JH, Goldstein SJ. Fractures of the articular processes of the cervical spine. AJR 1982; 139: 341–344.
4. Binet EF, Moro JJ, Marangola JP, Hodge CJ. Cervical spine tomography in trauma. Spine 1977; 2: 163–172.
5. Yetkin Z, Osborn AG, Giles DS, Haughton VM. Uncovertebral and facet joint dislocations in cervical articular pillar fractures: CT evaluation. AJNR 1985; 6: 633–637.

MRI

No studies have established any utility for MRI in the investigation of chronic neck pain. Its utility is entirely theoretical and speculative.

In principle, MRI is the best imaging technique that might be used to "clear" patients of serious disorders. Such disorders are rare, and should be evident on clinical grounds; but for practitioners concerned about occult lesions, in patients who are not recovering, MRI constitutes the best screening test. It has a high sensitivity and specificity for tumors, infections, and infiltrations of the epidural space. Although it does not resolve fractures well, it will nonetheless detect them. If better resolution of small fractures is of interest, CT can be directed at the segmental level implicated by MRI.

MRI is the only imaging modality that might be capable of detecting tears in the anterior anulus fibrosus, for it is the only modality that can resolve the soft tissues of the cervical spine. However, only one study has ever reported detecting rim lesions of the cervical discs.[1] Several other studies have failed to reproduce this observation.[2-6] Either these lesions are rare, or they are too small to be regularly detected by MRI using contemporary devices and protocols.

REFERENCES

1. Davis SJ, Teresi LM, Bradley WG, Ziemba M, Bloze AE. Cervical spine hyperextension injuries: MR findings. Radiology 1991; 180: 245–251.
2. Pettersson K, Hildingsson C, Toolanen G, Fagerlund M, Bjornebrink J. MRI and neurology in acute whiplash trauma. Acta Orthop Scand 1994; 65: 525–528.
3. Fagerlund M, Bjornebrink J, Pettersson K, Hildingsson C. MRI in acute phase of whiplash injury. Eur Radiol 1995; 5: 297–301.

4. Borchgrevink GE, Smevik O, Nordby A, Rinck PA, Stiules TC, Lereim I. MR imaging and radiography of patients with cervical hyperextension-flexion injuries after car accidents. Acta Radiol 1995; 36: 425–428.

5. Ronnen HR, de Korte PJ, Brink PRG, van der Bijl HJ, Tonino AJ, Franke CL. Acute whiplash injury: is there a role for MR imaging? A prospective study of 100 patients. Radiology 1996; 201: 93–96.

6. Voyvodic F, Dolinis J, Moore VM et al. MRI of car occupants with whiplash injury. Neuroradiology 1997; 39: 25–40.

PHYSIOLOGICAL TESTS

Pain is a sensory experience. It cannot be photographed or X-rayed. Radiographs are diagnostic of pain only if the lesion imaged has previously been shown to correlate with pain. When that correlation has not been established, and cannot be assumed, *imaging cannot be used to diagnose pain*. That is the case for most of the putative causes of chronic neck pain.

Since pain is a physiological phenomenon it requires physiological tests for its detection. For chronic neck pain two such tests are available. These tests do not determine the *cause* of pain but they do serve to pinpoint its *source* (see Chapter 2). For academic purposes, or to satisfy curiosity, imaging can subsequently be applied to the structure found to be painful, in order to identify the causative lesion. For practical purposes, however, that step is superfluous, if the pain can be treated without determining the exact cause.

CERVICAL DISCOGRAPHY

Cervical discography is a diagnostic test used by some practitioners to pinpoint pain arising from an intervertebral disc of the cervical spine. The test is based on the premise that if the target disc is the source of pain then provoking it with a mechanical stimulus should reproduce the patient's pain. The stimulus used is an injection of contrast medium into the nucleus pulposus of the disc.

The test involves inserting a needle, under fluoroscopic guidance, into the disc suspected of being painful, and into adjacent discs that serve as controls (Figure 13.1). Once the needles have been placed, contrast medium is injected into the discs in order to stress them. The test is positive if stressing the disc reproduces the pain.

If the patient's accustomed pain is reproduced, the pain is described as being *concordant* with the patient's accustomed or familiar pain. Any other form of pain that is produced is described as *dissimilar* to the patient's pain. In these terms, the objective of discography is to *detect reproduction of concordant pain*. Any other form of pain is not diagnostic.

Validity

For discography to be specific, it must be shown that the target disc is painful but that other discs are not. Otherwise, the test does not distinguish from generalized hyperalgesia of the neck, in which everything appears to be painful. When two or more discs appear painful the diagnosis becomes more troublesome and demanding, for then it still needs to be shown that other discs and other structures in the neck are not painful.

A further dimension relates to the intensity of stimulation. False-positive responses to disc stimulation can arise if the threshold for reproduction of pain is set too low. A disc is not necessarily the source of a patient's pain if the pain that is reproduced is minor or trivial.

A formal study compared the responses to discography in asymptomatic volunteers and in patients with neck pain.[1] It found that the numerical pain rating of pain produced by discography in asymptomatic subjects was significantly lower ($P = 0.000$) than that in patients with neck pain (Figure 13.2). It was unusual for volunteers to report pain greater than 5, and never greater than 6, on a 10-point numerical pain rating scale. Accordingly, the authors recommended an operational criterion that: the patient must rate the intensity *of the pain that is reproduced* as at least 7. The emphasis here is not on the intensity of the patient's baseline pain score, or by how much disc stimulation increases that pain. It is how intensely the patient rates the *evoked pain*. This criterion guards against diagnosing as positive a disc that is only moderately painful, but which could nevertheless be an asymptomatic disc.

Provocation of a cervical intervertebral disc may appear positive in spinal segments where other elements are the actual source of pain. This principle was demonstrated by a study that performed both discography and zygapophysial joint blocks at the same segments in a sample of patients with neck pain.[2] A false-positive response to discography was defined as one in which the disc was painful but anesthetizing the zygapophysial joints of the same segment completely relieved the patient of their pain. Such a response is incompatible with the disc being the primary source of pain, if a pain-source at all. The zygapophysial joints do not share a nerve supply with the discs. Therefore, anesthetizing the zygapophysial joints should not relieve discogenic pain. It relieves only zygapophysial joint pain. The implication is that if discography is positive in a patient whose pain can be relieved by zygapophysial joint blocks, the discography must be painful because it provoked pain not from the disc but from the zygapophysial joint.

In the 56 patients studied, discography was clearly positive in only 11 (20%). It was false-positive in

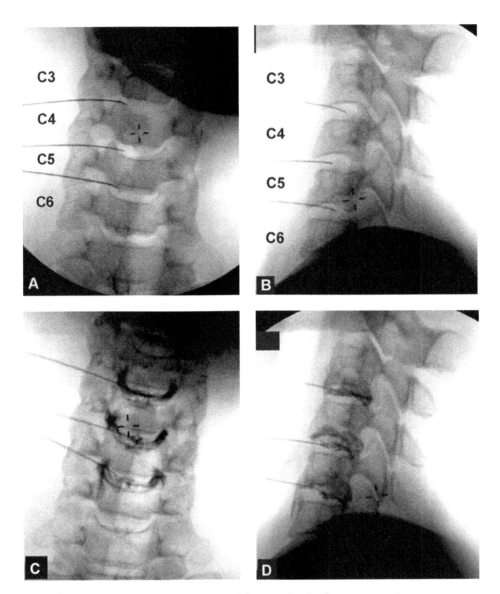

Figure 13.1 Radiographs illustrating cervical discography. (A,B) Anteroposterior and lateral views of needles placed in the nucleus pulposus of the C3–4, C4–5, and C5–6 intervertebral discs. (C,D) The appearance of the discs after injection of contrast medium. Reproduced from the practice guidelines for cervical disc stimulation of the International Spine Intervention Society.[3]

23 patients (41%) whose pain was relieved by zygapophysial joint blocks (Table 13.1). An alternative analysis revealed that of the 34 patients in whom discography appeared to be positive, it was false-positive in 23. This yields a false-positive rate of 68%, unless zygapophysial joint pain is first excluded, before undertaking cervical discography.

In order to maximize the specificity of cervical discography, this investigation should be conducted in manner so as to reduce, if not eliminate, the possibility of false-positive responses. To that end the International Spine Intervention Society recommended the following

operational criteria[3] (for the diagnosis of cervical discogenic pain, criteria A, B, C, and D must each be satisfied):

A. Discography has been correctly performed technically.
   This criterion guards against false-positive responses due to stimulation of the anulus fibrosus.
B. Cervical zygapophysial joint pain has been excluded at the segments being investigated.
   This criterion guards against false-positive responses due to concurrent zygapophysial

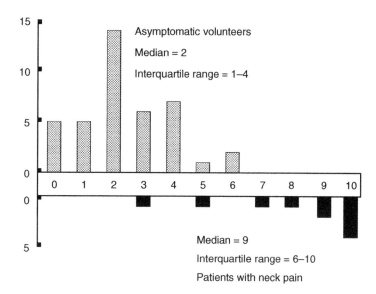

Figure 13.2 A histogram showing the number of asymptomatic patients and patients with neck pain who rated the evoked pain at the intensity indicated by the numerical pain rating scale. Based on Schellhas et al.[1]

joint pain. Unless this criterion is satisfied, the risk obtains of a 68% false-positive rate.

C. Stimulation of the target disc reproduces concordant pain.

This criterion is the primary objective of the test.

D. The pain that is reproduced is registered as at least 7 on a 10-point visual analogue or equivalent scale.

Criterion D ensures that normal and asymptomatic discs are not rated as positive because they are moderately painful.

E. Stimulation of adjacent discs does not reproduce the patient's pain.

This criterion ensures that the patient is not expressing hyperalgesia and a non-specific response to stimulation in the neck. It implies that, by definition, single-level discography cannot be valid, for single-level studies lack anatomical controls to show that adjacent levels are not symptomatic.

Discographers have been accustomed to investigating typically the lowest three cervical levels (C4–5,

Table 13.1 A correlation table between responses to provocation discography and zygapophysial joint blocks in patients who had both procedures at the segments indicated. Based on Bogduk and Aprill[2]

		Disc				
		Positive			**Negative**	
	Positive	C3–4:	2		C3–4:	1
		C4–5:	5		C4–5:	5
		C5–6:	4	=11	C5–6:	4	= 13
Zygapophysial joint					C6–7:	2
					C5–6,6–7:	1
	Negative	C3–4:	6		C3–4:	1
		C4–5:	3		C4–5:	4
		C5–6:	14	=23	C5–6:	1	= 9
					C4–5,5–6:	1
					C5–6,6–7:	2

C5–6, C6–7), and finding perhaps one or two of these levels to be positive, with the remaining levels serving as asymptomatic controls. A study has warned that this pattern of investigation may yield illusory results.

Grubb and Kelly[4] reviewed the responses to cervical discography in 173 patients. Where technically possible they investigated all levels from C2–3 to C6–7 in every patient. Levels obstructed by osteophytes or other anatomical impediments were omitted.

They found that, if all segmental levels are studied:

- single-level positive responses were uncommon (25%) (Table 13.2)
- three or more levels were usually positive
- discs at C3–4 are just as likely to be positive as discs at C4–5 and C5–6 (Table 13.3)
- discs at C2–3 were as likely to be positive as at C6–7.

These observations show that if studies are restricted to just the lower three levels, the investigation

Table 13.2 The incidence and pattern of distribution of positive responses to cervical discography when all segmental levels are studied in every patient. Based on Grubb and Kelly.[4] The dots indicate the levels tested. The black dots indicate levels found positive

Pattern	C2–3	C3–4	C4–5	C5–6	C6–7	C7–T1	Number of cases
One level positive N = 37	●	○	○	○	○	○	3
	○	●	○	○	○	○	7
	○	○	●	○	○	○	7
	○	○	○	●	○	○	13
	○	○	○	○	●	○	6
	○	○	○	○	○	●	1
Two levels positive N = 31	●	●	○	○	○	○	2
	●	○	●	○	○	○	1
	○	●	●	○	○	○	6
	○	●	○	●	○	○	5
	○	●	○	○	●	○	5
	○	○	●	●	○	○	4
	○	○	●	○	●	○	4
	○	○	○	●	●	○	4
Three levels positive N = 38	●	●	●	○	○	○	6
	●	●	○	●	○	○	1
	●	●	○	○	●	○	1
	●	○	●	●	○	○	1
	●	○	●	○	●	○	1
	○	●	●	●	○	○	12
	○	●	●	○	●	○	4
	○	●	●	○	○	●	1
	○	●	○	●	●	○	2
	○	○	●	●	●	○	9
Four levels positive N = 25	●	●	●	●	○	○	9
	●	●	●	○	●	○	3
	●	●	○	●	●	○	1
	●	○	●	●	●	○	1
	○	●	●	●	●	○	10
	○	●	●	●	○	●	1
Five levels positive	●	●	●	●	●	○	17
Six levels positive	●	●	●	●	●	●	1

Table 13.3 The prevalence and relative distribution of positive response to cervical discography, by segmental level, when all levels are studied in every patient. Based on Grubb and Kelly[4]

Discs studied		Discs found positive		Proportion of positive discs
Level	N	N	%	
C2–3	156	48	30	0.12
C3–4	168	94	55	0.24
C4–5	164	98	58	0.24
C5–6	152	91	55	0.23
C6–7	146	69	45	0.17
C7–T1	21	4	17	0.01

underestimates the number and location of positive levels.[2] If the investigations are extended to include higher levels, additional positive levels are likely to be encountered. Some 36% of positive discs occur at C2–3 and C3–4 (Table 13.3). Failing to study these levels conveniently avoids these additional positive responses, and renders the assessment of the patient either incomplete or confounded.

Although positive responses may be found at C4–5, C5–6, or C6–7, when just these levels are studied, the diagnosis, in effect, may be false-negative for having failed to detect positive discs at higher levels. The false-negative rate in that event is 36%. Simultaneously, the diagnosis of a positive disc at C4–5, C5–6, or both may be false-positive if, discs at C2–3 and C3–4 are also positive but have not been studied. What may appear to be a discrete diagnosis of positive discs at C4–5 and C5–6 (with a negative control at C6–7) may be wrong if discs at C2–3 and C3–4 are also positive. Although C4–5 and C5–6 discs were positive in 26 cases, in only four cases were they the only positive levels. In 13 cases either the C2–3 or the C3–4 disc was also positive; and in nine cases both C2–3 and C3–4 were positive (Table 13.2).

Unless and until refuted, these observations indicate that cervical discography is an incomplete and potentially flawed investigation if all segmental levels are not studied.

Although the study of Grubb and Kelly[4] invites that all cervical levels should be studied in every patient with neck pain, this may not always be practical. In particular, discography at C2–3 may be difficult and hazardous, and patients may find five-level discography a demanding procedure. A tension, therefore, arises

between the habit of routinely studying just three levels and the demand to study all levels. The International Spine Intervention Society proposed that whenever technically possible, cervical discography should be performed at four levels, in order to optimize the validity of the investigation; in patients with lower cervical pain, the C2–3 segment can be omitted, on the grounds that this segment is unlikely to be responsible for lower neck pain; and the C2–3 segment should be included only if the patient has headache as a major symptom, on the grounds that this segment is often positive in patients with headache.

Utility

Cervical discography has diagnostic utility if it provides an unequivocal diagnosis of cervical discogenic pain. Doing so protects patients from a futile pursuit of a diagnosis by other means.

The therapeutic utility of cervical discography rests on claims by surgeons that discography helps them select (and avoid) segmental levels that should be fused, in the treatment of neck pain; and that using discography improves outcomes.[5,6,7] These claims, however, are based only on observational studies. They have not been tested in a rigorous, controlled fashion.

However, cervical discography also has therapeutic utility in a negative sense. Finding multiple levels to be positive usually precludes surgical intervention. Cervical discography thus protects patients from undergoing unnecessary and unjustified surgery. In this regard, Grubb and Kelly[4] reported that only about 10% of their 173 patients underwent surgery after being investigated by cervical discography.

Prevalence

Despite the popularity of cervical discography as a diagnostic procedure, particularly among surgeons, the prevalence of cervical discogenic pain has not been formally studied and established. No population studies have determined what proportion of patients who present with neck pain have the cervical discs as the confirmed source of their pain. Some practitioners might believe that the discs are commonly the source of pain, but the available epidemiological data show that other conditions are substantially more common (q.v.).

REFERENCES

1. Schellhas KP, Smith MD, Gundry CR, Pollei SR. Cervical discogenic pain: prospective correlation of magnetic resonance imaging and discography in asymptomatic subjects and pain sufferers. Spine 1996; 21: 300–312.
2. Bogduk N, Aprill C. On the nature of neck pain, discography and cervical zygapophysial joint blocks. Pain 1993; 54: 213–217.
3. International Spine Intervention Society. Cervical Disc Stimulation. In: Bogduk N (ed). Practice Guidelines for Spinal Diagnostic and Treatment Procedures. International Spine Intervention Society, San Francisco, 2004: 95–111.
4. Grubb SA, Kelly CK. Cervical discography: clinical implications from 12 years of experience. Spine 2000, 25: 1382–1389.
5. Kikuchi S, Macnab I, Moreau P. Localisation of the level of symptomatic cervical disc degeneration. J Bone Joint Surg 1981; 63B: 272–277.
6. Whitecloud TS, Seago RA. Cervical discogenic syndrome: results of operative intervention in patients with positive discography. Spine 1987; 12: 313–316.
7. Garvey TA, Transfeldt EE, Malcolm JR, Kos P. Outcome of anterior cervical discectomy and fusion as perceived by patients treated for dominant axial-mechanical cervical spine pain. Spine 2002; 27: 1887–1894.

MEDIAL BRANCH BLOCKS

Medial branch blocks are a test for pain stemming from the cervical zygapophysial joints. They are based on the premise that if a patient's pain arises from a particular joint, then anesthetizing that joint should completely relieve their pain.

The cervical zygapophysial joints are innervated by the medial branches of the cervical dorsal rami.[1] Each joint receives articular branches from the nerve above and the nerve below the joint (Figure 13.3). Those nerves have the same segmental numbers as the joint. Each nerve crosses the middle of the ipsisegmental articular pillar. That point constitutes a suitable target point for blocks of the nerve.

The blocks are performed under fluoroscopic guidance. A needle is passed though the skin and muscles of the lateral neck until it reaches the midpoint of the articular pillar (Figure 13.4). At that point 0.3 ml of

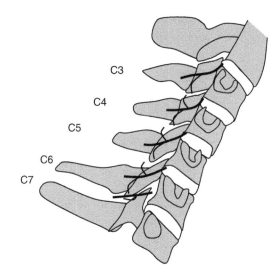

Figure 13.3 A sketch of the medial branches of the cervical dorsal rami and their articular branches to the cervical zygapophysial joints.

local anesthetic is injected in order to anesthetize the nerve. To completely block a given joint, both of the two nerves that innervate it must be anesthetized.

Validity

Cervical medial branch blocks are the most rigorously studied and validated diagnostic procedure for neck pain. They have been shown to have face validity, construct validity, and predictive validity. No other diagnostic test for neck pain has been shown to have these properties.

Face validity is the extent to which a test actually does what it is intended to do, in an anatomical and physiological sense. For cervical medial branch blocks, this was established by injecting contrast medium at the target points to test where the injectate spreads. The study showed that injectate concentrates at the target point for the target nerve, but does not spread to other structures, which if anesthetized might confound the result of the block.[2] The injectate does not spread to other nerves or to the spinal nerves, nor does it indiscriminately anesthetize the posterior neck muscles.

Construct validity is the measure of the extent to which the test correctly distinguishes patients who have the condition from those who do not. Three studies have addressed this issue for cervical medial branch blocks. The first showed that single blocks have an unacceptably high false-positive rate.[3] Therefore, to be valid, all blocks must be controlled.

Suitable controls are either placebo controls or comparative local anesthetic blocks. Placebo controls are appropriate for academic studies but are cumbersome in clinical practice because they require three

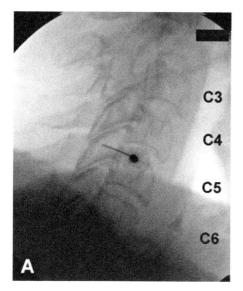
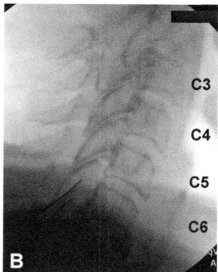

Figure 13.4 Lateral radiographs of the cervical spine showing needles in place for cervical medial branch blocks to anesthetize the C5–6 zygapophysial joint. (**A**) C5 medial branch block. (**B**) C6 medial branch block.

blocks to be conducted.[4,5,6] More practical are comparative local anesthetic blocks, in which different agents are administered on separate occasions. The response is positive if the patient has short-lived relief when a short-acting agent is used, but long-lasting relief when a long-acting agent is used.[4,5,6]

A study using comparative blocks used statistical arguments to show that positive responses were extremely unlikely to be false-positive, and were therefore valid.[7] That conclusion was verified by a study in which responses to comparative blocks were compared with those to placebo-controlled blocks.[8] Under those conditions, comparative blocks have a sensitivity of 86% and a specificity of 65%, which is sufficient for most clinical purposes. If greater certainty in the diagnosis is required, placebo controls should be used.[8]

The predictive validity of a test, also known as its therapeutic utility, is the extent to which it predicts successful outcome from the ensuing treatment. In this regard, a positive response to cervical medial branch blocks has been shown to predict successful outcomes from cervical medial branch neurotomy.[9,10,11] Comparative blocks and placebo-controlled blocks are equally powerful in this regard.[9,10,11]

Prevalence

Cervical medial branch blocks have been used in population studies to determine how often patients have chronic neck pain that stems from the cervical zygapophysial joints. The first study showed that the prevalence of zygapophysial joint pain was 54% (95% CI: 40–68%) in a sample of patients with chronic neck

pain after whiplash.[12] A subsequent study established a prevalence of 60% (95% CI: 46–73%).[13] Among drivers involved in high-speed collisions, the prevalence was as high as 74% (95% CI: 65–83%).[14] Other studies of patients with neck pain, not restricted to those with whiplash, have confirmed this pattern. In a rehabilitation practice, the prevalence of cervical zygapophysial joint pain was at least 36% (27–45%).[15] In a pain clinic it was 60%.[16]

Collectively, these data indicate that cervical zygapophysial joint pain is the single most common basis for chronic neck pain. It accounts for over 50% of patients. No other condition rivals this prevalence. For no other condition is the prevalence known. In effect, cervical zygapophysial joint pain is the only validated diagnosis of chronic neck pain.

HEADACHE

Cervical discography and cervical medial branch blocks have been used in the diagnosis of patients with neck pain and headache. The application and results of those tests are described in Chapter 23, in the context of cervicogenic headache.

OTHER TESTS

No other tests have been developed and validated for the diagnosis of chronic neck pain. Although some practitioners might believe that muscles or ligaments might be the source of pain, they have not provided tests capable of categorically attributing the pain to these sources.

Tests of muscle function, which determine weakness, imbalance, or other abnormalities, are not tests of the source of pain. Therefore, they are not diagnostic tests.

REFERENCES

1. Bogduk N. The clinical anatomy of the cervical dorsal rami. Spine 1982; 7: 319–330.
2. Barnsley L, Bogduk N. Medial branch blocks are specific for the diagnosis of cervical zygapophysial joint pain. Reg Anesth 1993; 18: 343–350.
3. Barnsley L, Lord S, Wallis B, Bogduk N. False-positive rates of cervical zygapophysial joint blocks. Clin J Pain 1993; 9: 124–130.
4. Bogduk N, Lord SM. Cervical zygapophysial joint pain. Neurosurg Quart 1998; 8: 107–117.
5. Bogduk N. Diagnostic nerve blocks in chronic pain. Best Pract Res Clin Anaesthesiol 2002: 16: 565–578.
6. International Spine Intervention Society. Cervical medial branch blocks. In: Bogduk N (ed). Practice Guidelines: Spinal Diagnostic and Treatment Procedures. International Spine Intervention Society, San Francisco, 2004: 112–137.
7. Barnsley L, Lord S, Bogduk N. Comparative local anaesthetic blocks in the diagnosis of cervical zygapophysial joints pain. Pain 1993; 55: 99–106.
8. Lord SM, Barnsley L, Bogduk N. The utility of comparative local anaesthetic blocks versus placebo-controlled blocks for the diagnosis of cervical zygapophysial joint pain. Clin J Pain 1995; 11: 208–213.
9. Lord SM, Barnsley L, Wallis BJ, McDonald GJ, Bogduk N. Percutaneous radio-frequency neurotomy for chronic cervical zygapophysial-joint pain. N Engl J Med 1996; 335: 1721–1726.
10. McDonald G, Lord SM, Bogduk N. Long-term follow-up of patients treated with cervical radiofrequency neurotomy for chronic neck pain. Neurosurgery 1999; 45: 61–68.
11. Lord SM, McDonald GJ, Bogduk N. Percutaneous radiofrequency neurotomy of the cervical medial branches: a validated treatment for cervical zygapophysial joint pain. Neurosurg Quart 1998; 8: 288–308.
12. Barnsley L, Lord SM, Wallis BJ, Bogduk N. The prevalence of chronic cervical zygapophysial joint pain after whiplash. Spine 1995; 20: 20–26.
13. Lord S, Barnsley L, Wallis BJ, Bogduk N. Chronic cervical zygapophysial joint pain after whiplash: a placebo-controlled prevalence study. Spine 1996; 21: 1737–1745.
14. Gibson T, Bogduk N, Macpherson J, McIntosh A. Crash characteristics of whiplash associated chronic neck pain. J Musculoskelet Pain 2000; 8: 87–95.
15. Speldewinde GC, Bashford GM, Davidson IR. Diagnostic cervical zygapophysial joint blocks for chronic cervical pain. Med J Aust 2001; 174: 174–176.
16. Manchikanti L, Singh V, Rivera J, Pampati V. Prevalence of cervical facet joint pain in chronic neck pain. Pain Physician 2002; 5: 243–249.

CHAPTER 14

Chronic neck pain: assessment

A practitioner may encounter a patient who presents for the first time with chronic neck pain, or the patient may be one of the practitioner's own patients whose pain has persisted since its acute phase. Those differences do not affect the basic principles of assessment. What differs is only the time required for the initial phases of assessment. If the practitioner is already familiar with the patient, less time will be required to obtain the history.

The cardinal steps in the assessment are provided in the form of an algorithm in Figure 14.1. The critical first step is to obtain a history. Physical examination will be of little diagnostic value, but should not be omitted. The assessment hinges on screening for red flags. Thereafter, a psychological assessment should be included, before proceeding to management.

HISTORY

There is a short component and a long component to obtaining the history. The short component pertains to screening for red flag indicators. For this purpose, the checklist recommended for acute neck pain (Chapter 5) can be used (Figure 14.2). If the checklist prompts any positive responses, appropriate medical action should be taken to explore the possibility of a serious cause of pain suggested by the response.

EXAMINATION

Physical examination has no greater reliability or validity in patients with chronic neck pain than it does for patients with acute neck pain (Chapter 6). As a rule it will not provide a diagnosis. Palpation may reveal tenderness; range of motion may be restricted; but neither of these features is diagnostic.

Nevertheless, physical examination complements taking a history with respect to screening for red flags. The patient should be examined for signs of rare disorders (e.g. pigmentation in von Recklinghausen's disease). If the patient has no neurological symptoms they should undergo a brief neurological examination in order to exclude major neurological signs. This should cover sensation and power in all four limbs.

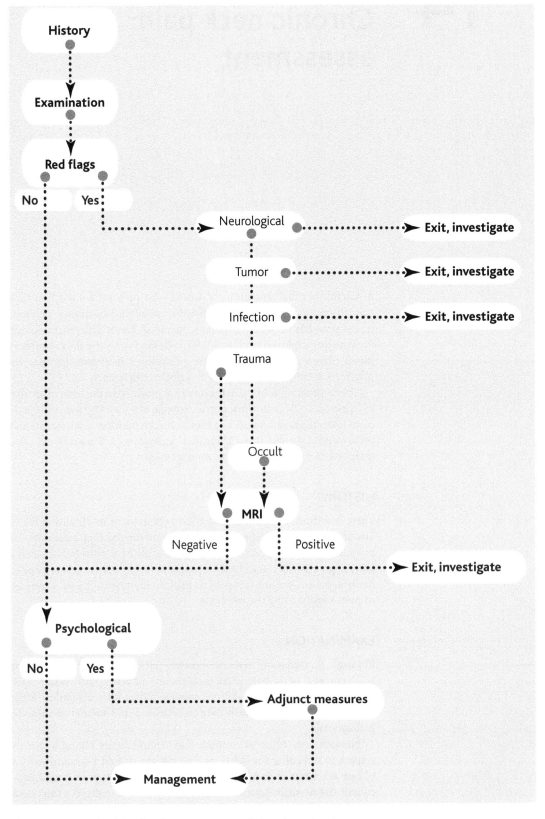

Figure 14.1 An algorithm for the management of chronic neck pain.

Name:			Neck Pain					
D.O.B			M.R.N.					
Trauma	Y	N	**Neurological**			**Endocrine**		
Fever	Y	N	Symptoms/signs	Y	N	Corticosteroids	Y	N
Night sweats	Y	N	Cerebrovascular	Y	N	Diabetes	Y	N
Recent surgery	Y	N	Vomiting	Y	N	Hyperparathyroid	Y	N
Catheterization	Y	N	**Cardiovascular**			**GIT**		
Venipuncture	Y	N	Risk factors	Y	N	Dysphagia	Y	N
Illicit drug use	Y	N	Anticoagulants	Y	N	**Musculoskeletal**		
Immunosuppression	Y	N	**Urinary**			Pain elsewhere	Y	N
Awkward posture	Y	N	UTI	Y	N	**Skin**		
Manipulation	Y	N	Hematuria	Y	N	Infections	Y	N
History of cancer	Y	N	Retention	Y	N	Rashes	Y	N
Weight loss	Y	N	**Reproductive**			**Respiratory**		
Exotic exposure	Y	N	Uterine	Y	N	Cough	Y	N
(Overseas) travel	Y	N	Breast	Y	N	**Signature:**		
Comments								
						Date:		

Figure 14.2 A checklist for red flag clinical indicators for neck pain, suitable for inclusion in medical records.

RED FLAGS

Patients with neurological symptoms, or with risk factors for infection, or with a suggestion of a tumor leave the algorithm, for they no longer have neck pain as their cardinal presenting feature. They have an indication of a possible serious cause of pain, which should be investigated irrespective of their neck pain.

For patients with a history of trauma to the neck or head, consideration should be given to the possibility of a fracture that has previously been missed. In such patients, radiography and CT are the least efficient investigations (Chapter 13). Radiography lacks sensitivity for small fractures, and CT cannot be used to screen the entire cervical spine for missed fractures. Similar comments apply to screening for occult lesions, i.e. serious conditions that are not manifest clinically. Unless the practitioner knows where to look, CT is not a suitable screening test.

Both for missed fractures and for occult lesions, MRI is the best screening test. It provides a complete view of the entire cervical spine without radiation exposure. It has good sensitivity and specificity for occult tumors and infections. It resolves fractures poorly but does not miss them. If a fracture is detected, CT can be used as a supplementary investigation to resolve the fracture better, if required.

If MRI detects a fracture or an occult lesion, the patient leaves the algorithm. Their further management is dictated by what is required for the lesion detected.

Degenerative disc disease, bulging discs, or osteoarthritis might be detected on MRI, but these are not diagnostic of the cause of pain. As in patients with acute neck pain, they are no more than normal age changes (Chapters 4 and 7).

If MRI is normal, the patient re-enters the algorithm as if they were a patient with no red flag indicators. In this regard, note that MRI is not advocated as a routine screening test. It is a loop in the algorithm precipitated by a red flag in the history. If there is no red flag, MRI is neither warranted nor justified.

PSYCHOLOGICAL ASSESSMENT

Psychological assessment of patients with chronic neck pain is a vexatious issue both academically and practically. Psychosocial factors have been found to be important determinants of chronicity in patients with low back pain. Therefore, psychological assessment of patients with back pain is regarded as paramount.

Some experts might maintain that the same applies for patients with chronic neck pain. However, evidence has not been published that psychosocial factors are as critical for neck pain as they are for back pain. The available evidence indicates that personal psychological factors are weak determinants of neck pain, and that the only psychosocial factors of possible significance are occupational in nature (Chapter 4). Nor have any formal psychometric tests, suitable for use outside research settings, been shown to be helpful in the management of chronic neck pain.

Nevertheless, the patient's psychosocial domain should not be ignored or neglected. In assessing this domain, the practitioner is not looking for a psychological cause for the patient's pain, for none can be legitimately and validly diagnosed. Rather, the practitioner is looking for additional components of the patient's overall problem, some of which may be amenable to parallel intervention.

These components can be detected, initially, in course of taking a conventional history. As the patient relates the history, the practitioner can notice particular elements. If required, the practitioner can explore particular issues as they arise. Sometimes, an additional consultation may be required to explore issues raised, or to check for issues not raised in the history.

The target issues may be: the level of distress of the patient and their perceived reasons for that distress; beliefs about the cause of their pain and its implications; concerns about their ability to work; concerns about medicolegal matters, if they apply. The practitioner should gain an impression about how the patient spends their day; why they are not working; or if they are working, what their circumstances at work are.

ADDITIONAL MEASURES

If psychosocial factors are identified, these invite management just as much as the neck pain does. The practitioner may elect to pursue management according to their own expertise, experience and confidence, or they may enlist the help of a colleague who specializes in this arena. In this regard, the target issues are not ones that are directly related to the pain. Those are addressed separately under Management (see later).

While not limited to the following, examples of what might require collateral management include:

- beliefs about the cause of pain and its significance
- realistic expectations of finding a diagnosis and/or a "cure"
- financial security
- the ability to work
- relationships at work
- the ability to maintain activities of daily living, despite the pain, or in a manner that least aggravates the pain
- understanding the compensation system, if one is involved.

Patients with whiplash injuries do not exhibit any particular or diagnostic psychiatric features. In terms of psychological profile, they do not differ substantially from patients who suffer other injuries.[1] What they do express, however, is anger at being an innocent victim in a frightening accident, subsequently subject to slowly progressing litigation.[1] Unless these issues are addressed and resolved in the course of management, the risk obtains that patients will retain their symptoms for as long as they are not acknowledged as innocent victims.

REFERENCE

1. Mayou R, Bryant B. Psychiatry of whiplash neck injury. Brit J Psychiat 2002; 180: 441–448.

MANAGEMENT

Pivotal to the management of the pain with which the patient presents is the question of investigation. The decision pertains not only to whether or not investigations are undertaken and which to undertake; it also predicates treatment. Precision investigations may provide for precision treatment. Not undertaking investigations limits the treatment options.

Investigations

Conventional medical imaging is highly unlikely to be diagnostic of the cause of chronic neck pain (Chapter 13). Plain radiography and CT are neither helpful nor reassuring. A normal film does not mean that there is nothing wrong. As a screening test, to clear patients of any missed serious diagnosis, MRI is the best investigation (Chapter 13).

Physiological tests are the only available means of establishing a diagnosis in patients with chronic neck pain (Chapter 13). Discography can determine if intervertebral discs are the source of pain. Medial branch blocks can determine if zygapophysial joints are the source.

Whether or not discography should be undertaken is a contentious issue. Cervical discography has unproven therapeutic utility. Cervical fusion is the only treatment currently available for patients with discogenic pain. One contention is that discography should be undertaken only if both patient and practitioner are prepared to pursue the surgical option. If they are not, then discography is not indicated. On the other hand, discography can nevertheless be justified on other grounds. Firstly, it may have negative predictive value. Finding multiple symptomatic discs constitutes a contraindication for surgery (Chapter 13). Such a result, therefore, may protect patients from unnecessary, futile surgery. Secondly, it may be satisfying to establish that a patient does have discogenic pain, even though surgery is not being entertained. Making such a diagnosis protects the patient from continuing to pursue a diagnosis that will be elusive by other means. Meanwhile, with a diagnosis having been made, the patient may derive some consolation from knowing that a proven treatment for their condition might become available in the future.

The situation is different for cervical medial branch blocks. Not only do these blocks have diagnostic utility (i.e. they pinpoint the source of pain), they also have therapeutic utility. Zygapophysial joint pain can be treated.

If investigations are not undertaken these options do not arise. Without a diagnosis the patient and the practitioner are limited to less than a handful of tested, let alone proven, interventions.

Treatment

The evidence concerning the treatment of chronic neck pain is detailed in Chapter 15. It transpires that there are very few proven treatments. Much of what is practiced is without any published foundation. Some interventions are not even based on descriptive studies.

Chronic neck pain: treatment

KEY POINTS

For the treatment of chronic neck pain:

- Controlled trials have not shown collars, TENS, traction, or multimodal therapy to be effective.

- Magnetic necklaces are no more effective than placebo.

- Acupuncture is no more effective than placebo.

- Injections of botulinum toxin or corticosteroids are not effective.

- The evidence shows no efficacy for manipulative therapy.

- Conventional physiotherapy has little beneficial effect, and is barely more effective than brief counseling.

- Multidisciplinary therapy appears to be helpful for behavioral features, although not for the relief of pain.

- Exercises seem to be the best commonly available treatment, but are not curative.

- The effectiveness of anterior cervical fusion or disc replacement remains contentious.

Percutaneous radiofrequency neurotomy for cervical zygapophysial joint pain:

- is the only treatment that has been validated in a double-blind, placebo-controlled trial

  and

- is the only treatment that has been shown to provide complete relief of chronic neck pain.

For many treatments used for chronic neck pain, there is no published evidence of efficacy.[1–5] There have been no published trials to demonstrate the efficacy of collar, transcutaneous electrical nerve stimulation (TENS), traction, trigger point therapy, or multimodal therapy for chronic neck pain. There is no evidence that drugs of any kind are an effective treatment for chronic neck pain. Magnetic necklaces are no more effective than a placebo.[6] For those interventions for which controlled studies have been conducted, the evidence is negative, mixed, or short of compelling.

REFERENCES

1. Bogduk N. The neck. Baillière's Clinical Rheumatology 1999; 13: 261–285.
2. Bogduk N. Whiplash: why pay for something that does not work? J Musculoskelet Pain 2000; 8: 29–53.
3. Bogduk N. Cervical pain. In: Ashbury AK, McKhann GM, McDonald WI, Goadsby PJ, MacArthur JC (eds). Disease of the Nervous system: Clinical Neuroscience and Therapeutic Principles. Cambridge University Press, Cambridge, 2002: 742–759.
4. Bogduk N. Neck and arm pain. In: Aminoff MJ, Daroff RB (eds). Encyclopedia of the Neurological Sciences. Academic Press, Amsterdam, 2003, 3: 390–398.
5. Bogduk N. Neck pain and whiplash. In: Jensen TS, Wilson PR, Rice ASC. Clinical Pain Management: Chronic Pain. Arnold, London, 2003: 504–519.
6. Hong CZ, Lin JC, Bender LF, Schaeffer JN, Meltzer RJ, Causin P. Magnetic necklace: its therapeutic effectiveness on neck and shoulder pain. Arch Phys Med Rehab 1982; 63: 426–466.

ACUPUNCTURE

Studies of acupuncture for chronic neck pain have produced conflicting results. An early study found acupuncture to be more effective than no treatment.[1] A small study found it to be more effective than placebo.[2] One study found acupuncture to provide a modest reduction in pain but barely greater than that of sham acupuncture.[3] Another found a greater, but not significant, reduction in pain compared to placebo treatment.[4] Otherwise, several studies have shown no greater benefit from acupuncture than from physiotherapy,[5,6] sham acupuncture,[7,8] or placebo treatment.[9,10] One study found placebo treatment to be more effective than acupuncture.[11]

REFERENCES

1. Coan RM, Wong G, Coan PL. The acupuncture treatment of neck pain: a randomised controlled study. Am J Chin Med 1982; 9: 326—332.
2. Petrie JP, Langley GB. Acupuncture in the treatment of chronic cervical pain: a pilot study. Clin Exp Rheumatol 1983; 1: 333—335.
3. Birch S, Jamison RB. Controlled trial of Japanese acupuncture for chronic myofascial neck pain: assessment of

specific and non-specific effects of treatment. Clin J Pain 1998; 14: 248–255.
4. He D, Veiersted KB, Hostmark AT, Medbo JI. Effect of acupuncture treatment on chronic neck and shoulder pain in sedentary female workers: a 6-month and 3-year follow-up study. Pain 2004; 109: 299–307.
5. Loy TT. Treatment of cervical spondylosis: electroacupuncture versus physiotherapy. Med J Aust 1983; 2: 32–34.
6. David J, Modi S, Aluko AA, Robertshaw C, Farebrother J. Chronic neck pain: a comparison of acupuncture treatment and physiotherapy. Brit J Rheumatol 1998; 37: 1118–1122.
7. Thomas MM, Eriksson SV, Lundeberg T. A comparative study of diazepam and acupuncture in patients with osteoarthritis pain: a placebo controlled study. Am J Chin Med 1991; 19: 95–100.
8. Irnich D, Behrens N, Molzen H et al. Randomised trial of acupuncture compared with conventional massage and "sham" laser acupuncture for treatment of chronic neck pain. Brit Med J 2001; 322: 1–6.
9. Lewith GT, Machin D. A randomised trial to evaluate the effect of infra-red stimulation of local trigger points, versus placebo, on the pain caused by cervical osteoarthrosis. Acupuncture and Electrotherapeut Res Int J 1981; 6: 277–284.
10. Petrie JP, Hazleman BL. A controlled study of acupuncture in neck pain. Brit J Rheumatol 1986; 25: 271–275.
11. Thorsen H, Gam AN, Svensson BH et al. Low level laser therapy for myofascial pain in the neck and shoulder girdle: a double-blind cross-over study. Scand J Rheumatol 1992; 21: 139–142.

INJECTIONS

Injections of botulinum toxin are not effective for chronic neck pain.[1] One study found trigger point injections to be as effective as ultrasound treatment[2] but another found ultrasound to be no more effective than placebo treatment.[3] Intra-articular injections of corticosteroids are not effective for cervical zygapophysial joint pain.[4]

REFERENCES

1. Wheeler AH, Goolkasian P, Gretz SS. Botulinum toxin A for the treatment of chronic neck pain. Pain 2001; 94: 255–260.
2. Esenyel CZ, Caglar N, Aldemir T. Treatment of myofascial pain. Am J Phys Med Rehabil 2000; 79: 48–52
3. Gam AN, Warming S, Larsen LH et al. Treatment of myofascial trigger points with ultrasound combined with massage and exercise: a randomised controlled trial. Pain 1998; 77: 73–79.
4. Barnsley L, Lord SM, Wallis BJ, Bogduk N. Lack of effect of intraarticular corticosteroids for chronic pain in the cervical zygapophyseal joints. N Engl J Med 1994; 330: 1047–1050.

MANIPULATION

Although manipulative therapy is a commonly used treatment for chronic neck pain, there is little literature on its efficacy. Some studies assessed the outcomes of manipulation immediately after treatment,[1,2] at 1 week,[3,4] or at only 3 weeks[5] after treatment. Others have conducted longer follow-up.[6–9] One study enrolled patients with either back pain or neck pain, but the published data pertain only to back pain.[10,11] Nevertheless, reviewers have managed to obtain from the authors those data that pertain to the patients with neck pain.[12]

A systematic review[12] found no evidence of benefit from manipulative therapy or cervical mobilization for chronic neck pain. It concluded that:

- manipulation alone, utilizing one session, consistently showed evidence of *no benefit* when compared with a control or comparison group;[1,2,5] and
- manipulation in combination with mobilization showed *no evidence of benefit* when compared with a placebo, the combination of analgesics, anti-inflammatory medication and patient education, or the multimodal treatment combination of massage, exercise and physical medicine methods.[10,11]

A well-reported study, with long-term follow-up, showed that manipulation confers no greater benefit than intensive exercises or physiotherapy.[8] Another found that strengthening exercises were more beneficial than manipulative therapy.[6,7]

Collectively these data deny any utility of manual therapy for chronic neck pain. For acute neck pain, there is some support for manual therapy when used as part of a multimodal treatment program (Chapter 10). For chronic neck pain there is no evidence of an equivalent efficacy.[12]

REFERENCES

1. Cassidy JD, Lopes AA, Yong-Hing K. The immediate effects of manipulation versus mobilization on pain and range of motion in the cervical spine: a randomized controlled trial. J Manip Physiol Ther 1992; 15: 570–575.
2. Vernon HT, Aker P, Burns S, Viljakaanen S, Short L. Pressure pain threshold evaluation of the effect of spinal manipulation in the treatment of chornic neck pain: a pilot study. J Manip Physiol Ther 1990; 13: 13–16.
3. Brodin H. Cervical pain and mobilization. Int J Rehab Res 1984; 7: 190–191.
4. Brodin H. Cervical pain and mobilization. Man Med 1985; 2: 18–22.
5. Sloop PR, Smith DS, Goldenberg E, Dore C. Manipulation for chronic neck pain: a double-blind controlled study. Spine 1982; 7: 532–535.
6. Bronfort G, Evens R, Nelson B, Aker PD, Goldsmith CH, Vernon H. A randomized clinical trial of exercise and spinal manipulation for patients with chronic neck pain. Spine 2001; 26: 788–799.
7. Evans R, Bronfort G, Nelson B, Goldsmith CH. Two-year follow-up of a randomized clinical trial of spinal manipulation and two types of exercise for patients with chronic neck pain. Spine 2002; 27: 2383–2389.
8. Jordan A, Bendix T, Nielsen H, Hansen FR, Winkel A. Intensive training, physiotherapy, or manipulation for patients with chronic neck pain: a prospective, single-blinded, randomized clinical trial. Spine 1998; 23: 311–319.
9. Vasseljen O, Johansson BM, Wesgaard RH. The effect of pain reduction on perceived tension and EMG-recorded trapezius muscle activitiy in workers with shoulder and neck pain. Scand J Rehab Med 1995; 27: 243–252.
10. Koes BW, Bouter LM, van Mameren H et al. The effectiveness of manual therapy, physiotherapy, and treatment by the general practitioner for nonspecific back and neck complaints: a randomized clinical trial. Spine 1992; 17: 28–35.
11. Koes BW, Bouter LM, van Mameren H et al. Randomised clinical trial of manipulative therapy and physiotherapy for persistent back and neck complaints: results of one year follow-up. BMJ 1992; 304: 601–605.
12. Gross AR, Kay T, Hondras M et al. Manual therapy for mechanical neck disorders: a systematic review. Man Ther 2002; 7: 131–149.

PHYSIOTHERAPY

Whereas most studies of the treatment of chronic neck pain have focused on single interventions or set combinations of interventions, one has examined the efficacy of physiotherapy in a study in which therapists were free to apply whatever intervention they felt was indicated.[1] To various extents patients in the physiotherapy group received Maitland mobilization, McKenzie therapy, advice on posture, lifting, and lifestyle, electrotherapy, and to a lesser extent various other interventions. A comparison group underwent a brief intervention consisting of encouragement to return to normal activities through self-management.

At 3-months and 12-month follow-up, there were few differences in outcome between the two groups. Both exhibited small improvements in pain, ranging between 5 and 11 points on a 100-point scale. There were no differences at 3 months, but at 12 months the outcomes favored physiotherapy. In terms of physical and social functioning there were no differences between the groups at any time.

Two features are apparent from the results of this study. Firstly, physiotherapy is little more effective than a brief session of advice. Secondly, neither intervention has a clinically significant effect. Such improvements as were achieved were small on all outcome scales.

REFERENCE

1. Klaber Moffett JA, Jackson DA, Richmond S et al. Randomised trial of a brief physiotherapy intervention compared with usual physiotherapy for neck pain patients: outcomes and patients' preference. BMJ 2005; 330: 75–78.

MULTIDISCIPLINARY THERAPY

A systematic review found only two studies of multidisciplinary biopsychosocial rehabilitation for neck pain, neither of which provided evidence of efficacy.[1] A non-experimental study showed that multimodal cognitive-behavioral treatment achieved greater reductions in pain intensity in treated patients than in a non-treated comparison cohort, but the improvement amounted to no more than a reduction in pain intensity from 54 to 40 on a 100-point scale.[2]

An uncontrolled study showed that a multimodal behavioral and physical program could normalize somatic and cognitive complaints in a large proportion of patients, but reductions in pain were only modest.[3] The investigators did not report raw scores on various outcome measures. Instead they reported the proportion of patients that achieved scores, for each outcome measure, in what the investigators considered a healthy range (Table 15.1). These are the strongest available data on the efficacy of behavioral therapy for chronic neck pain. Without controls, the data are of limited value. Nevertheless, they are encouraging. They suggest that, for behavioral domains, behavioral therapy can help patients regain normal status.

REFERENCES

1. Karjalainen K, Malmivaara A, van Tulder M et al. Multidisciplinary biopsychosocial rehabilitation for neck and shoulder pain among working age adults: a systematic review with the framework of the Cochrane collaboration back review group. Spine 2001; 26: 174–181.
2. Jensen IB, Bodin L. Multimodal cognitive-behavioural treatment for workers with chronic spinal pain: a matched cohort study with an 18-months follow-up. Pain 1998; 76: 35–44.
3. Vendrig AA, van Akkerveeken PF, McWhorter KR. Results of a multimodal treatment program for patients with chronic symptoms after a whiplash injury of the neck. Spine 2000; 25: 2389–244.

EXERCISE

Exercises of various types have been the most extensively studied intervention for chronic neck pain. The outcomes reveal certain patterns (Table 15.2). On average, patients treated with exercises show improvements in pain scores. Depending on the study, and depending on the type of exercises, these improvements range between 25% and 75% reduction in pain. Exercises are as effective as manual therapy or physiotherapy.[2,4,5] Strengthening exercises are no more effective than endurance exercises.[7] Intensive exercises are more effective than light exercises[1] but not necessarily more effective than ordinary activity.[6] Special stabilizing exercises are not more effective than home exercises;[3] and are barely more

Table 15.1 The outcomes of a multimodal behavioral therapy program for chronic neck pain[3]

Domain	Proportion of patients within "healthy range" at 6 months
Pain < 10/100	46%
Disability	38%
Use of drugs	58%
Return to full work	65%
Return to some work	92%
No medical consumption	81%
Cognitive complaints	85%
Depression	96%

effective than heat treatment.[8] Outcomes are better if patients are instructed in the exercises.[3]

These data would support exercises to be the treatment of choice for chronic neck pain, from among the conventional interventions. However, exercises are not curative. Although they might reduce pain, they do not eliminate it.

REFERENCES

1. Randlov A, Ostergaard M, Manniche C et al. Intensive dynamic training for females with chronic neck/shoulder pain: a randomised controlled trial. Clin Rehabil 1998; 12: 200–210.
2. Jordan A, Bendix T, Nielsen H, Hansen FR, Host D, Winkel A. Intensive training, physiotherapy, or manipulation for patients with chronic neck pain: a prospective, single-blinded, randomised clinical trial. Spine 1998; 23: 311–319.
3. Taimela S, Takala EP, Asklof T, Seppala K, Parvainen S. Active treatment of chronic neck pain: a prospective randomised intervention. Spine 2000; 25: 1021–1027.
4. Bronfort G, Evans R, Nelson B, Aker PD, Goldsmith CH, Vernon H. A randomised clinical trial of exercise and spinal manipulation for patients with chronic neck pain. Spine 2001; 26: 788–799.
5. Evans R, Bronfort G, Nelson B, Goldsmith CH. Two-year follow-up of a randomised clinical trial of spinal manipulation and two types of exercise for patients with chronic neck pain. Spine 2002; 27: 2383–2389.
6. Viljanen M, Malmivaara A, Uitti J, Rinne M, Palmroos P, Lappala P. Effectiveness of dynamic muscle training, relaxation training, ordinary activity for chronic neck pain: randomised controlled trial. Brit Med J 2003; 327: 475.
7. Ylinen J, Takala EP, Nykanen M et al. Active neck muscle training in the treatment of chronic neck pain in women: a randomized controlled trial. JAMA 2003; 289: 2509–2516.
8. Chiu TTW, Lam THL, Hedley AJ. A randomised controlled trial on the efficacy of exercise for patients with chronic neck pain. Spine 2005; 30: E1–E7.

Table 15.2 Pain scores from studies of exercises for chronic neck pain

Study	Treatment	Pain scores				
		Baseline	3M	4M	6M	12M
Randlov et al.[1]	Intensive exercises	60			40	45
	Light exercises	60	50		60	60
Jordan et al.[2]	Intensive exercises	40		10		15
	Physiotherapy + manual therapy	40		10		20
	Manual therapy	43		15		15
Taimela et al.[3]	Multimodal stabilization exercises	43	22			
	Home exercises with instruction	31	23			No difference
	Home exercises written	40	39			
Bronfort et al.[4,5]	Manual therapy + exercises	57	30		30	31
	Exercises	57	25		30	30
	Manual therapy	57	37		36	37
Viljanen et al.[6]	Dynamic exercises	48	29		29	31
	Relaxation	48	29		30	33
	Ordinary activity	41	27		29	32
Ylinen et al.[7]	Strengthening exercises	50				18
	Endurance exercises	57				22
	Written advice Home stretching	58				34
Chiu et al.[8]	Dynamic strengthening	46			31	
	Infra-red heat	43			38	

ANTERIOR CERVICAL FUSION

There is an abundant literature describing the techniques for anterior cervical fusion. Some of the literature provides observational data on outcome.[1–11] Most, however, describe the treatment of patients with radicular pain, not chronic neck pain. Those studies that enrolled mixed samples of patients did not stratify their results according to the condition for which patients were treated. Therefore, it is not possible to extract data from these studies on the efficacy of fusion for neck pain.

Only three studies have provided data on the outcomes of fusion explicitly for patients with neck pain uncomplicated by radicular pain. None of these studies, however, was rigorous with respect to the assessment of outcomes, using measures normally expected of studies of pain.

The earliest study focused on the utility of cervical discography.[12] The authors mentioned that they obtained better outcomes in patients in whom they performed discography than in those they had previously treated without first using discography.

The second study also addressed the utility of discography in planning cervical fusion.[13] It reported that 10 (32%) of 34 patients had excellent results, and 13 (38%) had good results.

The most recent study[14] used patient satisfaction as the main outcome measure. In this regard, 82% of patients rated their outcome to be good, very good, or excellent. Some 57% of patients reported that their pain was much better after surgery, but only 10% were rendered free of pain. On average, disability improved from 59 to 31 on a 0–100 scale for the modified Oswestry disability index, and from 16 to 8 on a 0–25 modified Roland Morris disability index.

These reported data are consistent with the stated reputation of cervical fusion being an effective intervention. However, the available data are incomplete. It seems that only a small proportion of patients are rendered free of pain. It is not evident what proportion are successfully rehabilitated. Nor is it evident what proportion resumed normal activities of daily living, including work, or what proportion still required some form of continuing care.

REFERENCES

1. Smith GW, Robinson RA. The treatment of certain cervical spine disorders by anterior removal of the intervertebral disc and interbody fusion. J Bone Joint Surg 1958; 40A: 607–624.
2. Robinson RA, Walker AE, Ferlic DC, Wieking DK. The results of anterior interbody fusion for the cervical spine. J Bone Joint Surg 1962; 44A: 1569–1587.
3. Hirsch C, Wickbom I, Lidstrom A, Rosengren K. Cervical disc resection: a follow-up of myelographic and surgical procedure. J Bone Joint Surg 1964; 46A: 1811–1821.
4. De Plama AF, Subin DK. Study of the cervical syndrome. Clin Orthop 1965; 38: 135–142.
5. Dohn DF. Anterior interbody fusion for treatment of cervical-disk conditions. JAMA 1966; 197: 897–900.
6. Williams JL, Allen MB, Harkess JW. Late results of cervical diskectomy and interbody fusion: some factors influencing the results. J Bone Joint Surg 1968; 50A: 277–286.
7. Simmons EH, Bhalla SK. Anterior cervical diskectomy and fusion: a clinical and biomechanical study with eight-year follow-up. J Bone Joint Surg 1969; 51B: 225–237.
8. White AA, Southwick WO, DePonte RJ, Gainor JW, Hardy R. Relief of pain by anterior cercal-spine fusion for spondylosis. J Bone Joint Surg 1973; 55A: 525–534.
9. Green PWB. Anterior cervical fusion: a review of thirty-three patients with cervical disc degeneration. J Bone Joint Surg 1977; 59B: 236–240.
10. Clements DH, O'Leary PF. Anterior cervical diskectomy and fusion. Spine 1990; 15: 1023–1025.
11. Emery SE, Bolesta MJ, Banks MA, Jones PK. Robinson anterior cervical fusion: comparison of the standard and modified techniques. Spine 1994; 19: 660–663.
12. Kikuchi S, Macnab I, Moreau P. Localisation of the level of symptomatic cervical disc degeneration. J Bone Joint Surg 1981; 63B: 272–277.
13. Whitecloud TS, Seago RA. Cervical discogenic syndrome: results of operative intervention in patients with positive discography. Spine 1987; 12: 313–316.
14. Garvey TA, Transfeldt EE, Malcolm JR, Kos P. Outcome of anterior cervical diskectomy and fusion as perceived by patients treated for dominant axial-mechanical cervical spine pain. Spine 2002; 27: 1887–1894.

DISC REPLACEMENT

A side-effect of cervical fusion is loss of segmental mobility, with accelerated degeneration of adjacent segments.[1] Disc replacement is emerging as a means of avoiding these side-effects in the treatment of cervical disc disease. The theory is that a disc prosthesis maintains normal motion at the treated segments and at adjacent segments.

To date, disc replacement has been used to treat patients with cervical radiculopathy or myelopathy.[2,3]

No publications have reported its use for neck pain or somatic referred pain. It may become an option for the treatment of chronic neck pain.

REFERENCES

1. Albert TJ, Eichenbaum D. Goals of cervical disc replacement. Spine J 2004; 4: 292S–293S.
2. Anderson PA, Sasso RC, Rouleau JP, Carlson CS, Goffin J. The Bryan cervical disc: wear properties and early clinical results. Spine J 2004; 4: 303S–309S.
3. Pimenta L, McAfee PC, Cappuccino A, Bellera FP, Link HD. Clinical experience with the new artificial cervical PCM (Cervitech) disc. Spine J 2004; 4: 315S–321S.

RADIOFREQUENCY NEUROTOMY

The one treatment that has been shown to relieve neck pain completely is percutaneous radiofrequency medial branch neurotomy for proven cervical zygapophysial joint pain. The treatment involves carefully coagulating the medial branches of the dorsal rami that are responsible for mediating the patient's pain[1] (Figure 15.1). The singular indication is complete relief of pain following controlled diagnostic blocks of these nerves.

A placebo controlled trial showed that this is a valid procedure.[2] Complete relief of pain is achieved in some 70% of patients treated.[2,3,4] Errors in diagnosis account for the failures. Some patients have false-positive responses to diagnostic blocks, even when these are controlled. In other patients, neurotomy unmasks latent, or previously undiagnosed sources of pain, e.g. at adjacent segmental levels.

Follow-up studies have shown that relief after medial branch neurotomy lasts for a median period of

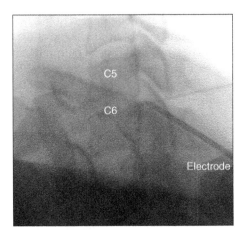

Figure 15.1 A lateral radiograph of the cervical spine, showing an electrode in place for radiofrequency neurotomy of a C6 medial branch, in the course of treatment of C5–6 zygapophysial joint pain.

between 270 and 400 days.[2,3,4] Pain recurs because the coagulated nerves regenerate but in that event, complete relief can be reinstated by repeating the procedure.[2,3,4] Outcomes are not demonstrably different between patients with legal claims and those without.[2,4,5]

Radiofrequency neurotomy is applicable to those 60% of patients with chronic neck pain who have positive responses to controlled medial branch blocks. Not only does radiofrequency neurotomy relieve pain, it also resolves psychological distress immediately that pain is relieved.[6] No other treatment for chronic neck pain has been shown to have these properties. An independent review reported that radiofrequency neurotomy sets a benchmark for the treatment of chronic neck pain.[7]

REFERENCES

1. Lord SM, Barnsley L, Bogduk N. Percutaneous radiofrequency neurotomy in the treatment of cervical zygapophysial joint pain: a caution. Neurosurgery 1995; 36: 732–739.

2. Lord SM, Barnsley L, Wallis BJ, McDonald GJ, Bogduk N. Percutaneous radio-frequency neurotomy for chronic cervical zygapophysial-joint pain. N Engl J Med 1996; 335: 1721–1726.

3. Lord SM, McDonald GJ, Bogduk N. Percutaneous radiofrequency neurotomy of the cervical medial branches: a validated treatment for cervical zygapophysial joint pain. Neurosurg Quart 1998; 8: 288–308.

4. McDonald G, Lord SM, Bogduk N. Long-term follow-up of patients treated with cervical radiofrequency neurotomy for chronic neck pain. Neurosurgery 1999; 45: 61–68.

5. Sapir DA, Gorup JM. Radiofrequency medial branch neurotomy in litigant and nonlitigant patients with cervical whiplash. Spine 2001; 26: E268–E273.

6. Wallis BJ, Lord SM, Bogduk N. Resolution of psychological distress of whiplash patients following treatment by radiofrequency neurotomy: a randomised, double-blind, placebo-controlled trial. Pain 1997; 73: 15–22.

7. Centre for Health Services and Policy Branch. Percutaneous radio-frequency neurotomy treatment of chronic cervical pain following whiplash injury. Vancouver, University of British Columbia, British Columbia Office of Health Technology Assessment 01:5T, 2001.

4 Mechanisms of whiplash

16 Whiplash: abridged summary

Not all patients who suffer a motor vehicle accident sustain an injury. Some individuals develop no symptoms, and the majority of those who do develop symptoms recover (Chapter 4). These epidemiological data suggest that the majority sustain no substantive or lasting injury. At most, perhaps, they suffer minor sprains of the neck muscles or ligaments.

A small proportion of victims, however, develop persistent symptoms, which warrant an explanation. Biomechanics and pathology studies have revealed what the underlying injuries and their mechanisms can be.

This chapter provides a succinct summary of the available evidence concerning the mechanisms of injury and the mechanisms of symptoms reported by patients with whiplash-associated neck pain. Readers interested in further information can consult Chapters 17 and 18.

BIOMECHANICS

Contrary to popular belief, whiplash is not a flexion-extension injury. Biomechanics studies have shown that whiplash is a compression injury. Following impact, the trunk is thrust upwards, against the inertia of the head. This causes a sigmoid deformation of the cervical spine. Within this deformation, lower cervical segments undergo an abnormal rotation into extension, during which the anterior anulus fibrosus is distracted and the zygapophysial joints are impacted.

Whether an injury occurs in a given case depends on the magnitude of impact, and the resistance to injury of the structures stressed. In experimental studies, normal volunteers develop symptoms following impacts at speeds greater than 10 km per hour.

PATHOLOGY

Pathology studies corroborate the lesions predicted by biomechanics studies. These encompass tears of the anterior anulus fibrosus, contusions of the intra-articular meniscoids of the zygapophysial joints, and fractures of the articular pillars or subchondral plates of these joints.

SYMPTOMS

Pain

The cardinal and characteristic symptom of whiplash is *neck pain*. This pain may be referred to the head or to the upper limb girdle. In patients with persistent pain, its cause can be understood in terms of the injuries that can befall the neck as a result of whiplash. Injuries of either the anulus fibrosus or the zygapophysial joints would readily cause neck pain and somatic referred pain.

There is nothing distinctive about the neck pain caused by whiplash. Its treatment is the same as that for idiopathic neck pain.

Other symptoms

A variety of other symptoms are often regarded as being caused by whiplash. They are reported by various proportions of patients, sometimes by only a small minority.

Paresthesiae, dizziness, and *visual disturbances* can be explained in terms of various secondary and reflex responses to pain. They do not necessarily imply injuries of the brain or peripheral nervous system.

Similarly, *cognitive impairments* are not necessarily a sign of brain damage. Disturbances in concentration and memory can be secondary to headache, or side-effects of drugs used to treat neck pain.

Back pain is a symptom reported by some 30–40% of patients who suffer whiplash-associated neck pain. Back pain in such patients has not been subjected to concerted study. It is not evident if there is a mechanism by which patients might injure their lumbar spine in a whiplash accident, or if the complaint of back pain represents no more than the prevalence of back pain in the community.

Tinnitus is the most vexatious symptom to explain. No models have been postulated to link tinnitus to neck pain. The only explanations that have been offered invoke some form of damage to the inner ear, as a result of whiplash.

17 Whiplash: mechanics of injury

KEY POINTS

- Whiplash is largely a compression injury, in which the trunk is forced upwards into the cervical spine.

- The cervical spine undergoes a sigmoid deformation.

- During the deformation, lower cervical segments undergo rotations about an abnormally located axis of rotation.

- The anterior anulus fibrosus of the disc is strained, and the zygapophysial joints are impacted.

- Injuries to the disc and zygapophysial joints predicted from biomechanics studies have been verified in post-mortem studies.

Whiplash is an event that occurs during a motor vehicle accident. Traditionally it is the motion suffered by the cervical spine during a rear-end motor vehicle collision. Modern usage, however, now includes the motions suffered during side-impact and front-end collisions. The cardinal feature of whiplash is that it is an inertial event. It explicitly does not encompass events in which a direct blow is sustained to the head or neck, be that from the roof, dashboard, or side wall of the vehicle. During whiplash, energy from the collision is transferred to the neck from the trunk (of the body), and the resultant motion of the cervical spine is produced when the inertia of the head reacts to this energy.

MECHANISMS

Modern studies have dispelled previous misconceptions about what happens during whiplash.[1] Whiplash does not involve flexion-extension injury,[2] acceleration-deceleration injury,[3] or cantilever injury[4] of the cervical spine.

Using high-speed photography, McConnell et al.[5] demonstrated what happens to the head, neck and trunk during experimental, rear-end whiplash in volunteers (Figure 17.1). Between 0 and 50 ms after impact, there is no response by the body. During this period the vehicle and seat absorb the

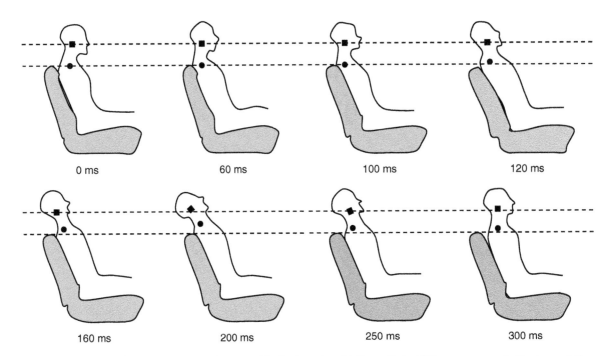

0 ms 60 ms 100 ms 120 ms

160 ms 200 ms 250 ms 300 ms

Figure 17.1 Whiplash motion as seen photographically, based on McConnell et al.[5] The square marks the base of the head. The round dot marks the base of the neck. The principal movement of whiplash is elevation of the base of the neck against the head.

impact forces. At 60 ms, the hips and lower trunk are thrust upward and forward. By 100 ms the upper trunk moves upward and forward. The upward movement compresses the cervical spine from below. The forward movement displaces the neck and trunk forward of the line of gravity of the head. As a result, by 120 ms, the center of gravity of the head starts to drop and causes the head to rotate backward. By 160 ms the torso pulls the base of the neck forward, and tension through the cervical spine draws the head forward. At about 250 ms the trunk and neck start to descend, and complete their descent by 300 ms. During this period the head continues forward, progressing slightly forward of the neutral, upright position, reaching its maximum forward excursion by 400 ms. Between 400 and 600 ms, the head moves backward slightly to restore its neutral position. At no time during this motion do the head and cervical spine exceed their normal, physiological range of motion.

Investigators studying cadavers subjected to whiplash have identified two kinematic phases.[6,7] Studies using high-speed cineradiography in volunteers have corroborated those observations.[8] Phase I occurs as the trunk is thrust upward and forward into the neck (Figure 17.2). During this phase, the cervical spine first undergoes a sigmoid deformation.[8,9,10] The lower segments extend while the upper segments flex. Subsequently, as the trunk proceeds forward and the head drops, the upper cervical segments extend. Phase II commences

once the entire cervical spine has extended. As the trunk and base of the neck drop, the head returns to its normal position over the base of the neck. There is no conspicuous 'flexion' movement. Phase II essentially involves only restitution of the original, resting position of the head and neck.

The extension of the lower cervical spine that occurs during phase I is not normal in nature. Normally, extension occurs around an axis of rotation located in the vertebral body of the vertebra below the moving

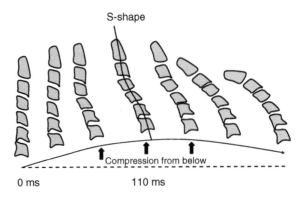

S-shape

Compression from below

0 ms 110 ms

Figure 17.2 A sketch of the radiographic appearance of the cervical spine during phase I of whiplash, based on Kaneoka et al.[8] The base of the neck rises. At about 110 ms after impact, the cervical spine is compressed into a sigmoid shape. Extension is completed as the base of the neck descends.

one[11] (Figure 17.3A). Under this condition, the moving vertebra translates backward as it rotates into extension. As it does so, its inferior articular facets glide virtually tangentially across the supporting superior articular facets.

During whiplash, the extension occurs about an abnormally located axis. It lies in the moving vertebra, not in the one below[8] (Figure 17.3B). This displacement of the axis indicates that the extension exclusively involves posterior sagittal rotation; there is no posterior translation of the vertebra. As a result of this abnormal motion, anteriorly the vertebral bodies are separated to an abnormal degree, while posteriorly, instead of gliding, the inferior articular processes chisel into the superior articular processes (Figure 17.4).

Within individual segments, therefore, abnormal motion can occur, even though the total range of motion of the neck remains within physiological limits. The extension of segments C6–7 and C7–T1 can exceed normal limits.[9,12] During phase I the zygapophysial joints undergo compression that exceeds physiological limits; and during phase II the anterior capsules of these joints are strained beyond normal limits.[7,13] In both instances, the abnormal strains are greater as the magnitude of impact increases. Meanwhile, strains in the anulus fibrosus can exceed normal limits.[6] At low accelerations, the strains are greatest in the C4–5 disc, but become abnormal also at C3–4, C5–6, and C6–7 as impact accelerations increase.

Collectively, the biomechanics studies predict a variety of possible injuries resulting from whiplash

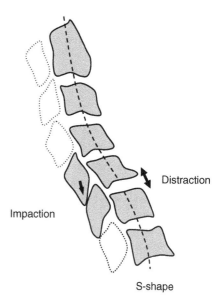

Figure 17.4 A sketch of the radiographic appearance of the cervical spine at about 110 ms after impact, based on Kaneoka et al.[8] The sigmoid deformation of the cervical spine causes abnormal rotation of the lower cervical segments, during which the anterior elements are distracted while the posterior elements are impacted.

kinematics (Figure 17.5). These include strain or avulsion of the anterior anulus fibrosus, strain of the zygapophysial joint capsules, and impaction injuries to the zygapophysial joints ranging from contusions to intra-articular meniscoids and resultant intra-articular hemorrhage, to subchondral and transarticular fractures. Whether or not these injuries occur depends on the magnitude of impact and the susceptibility or resistance to injury of the possible target structures.

For ethical reasons, all laboratory studies in normal volunteers have been conducted using low-speed collisions, typically between 2 and 10 km per hour. Even so, some of the subjects developed symptoms such as

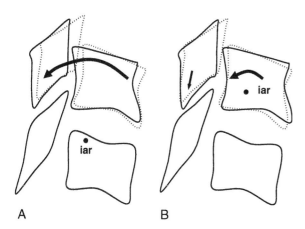

Figure 17.3 The motion of lower cervical spine segments about their instantaneous axis of rotation (iar). **(A)** Under normal conditions the axis lies in the lower vertebra, and the zygapophysial joints glide backward tangential to the superior articular process. **(B)** In whiplash, the axis lies in the moving vertebra, around a shorter radius, so that the inferior articular process chisels into the superior articular process.

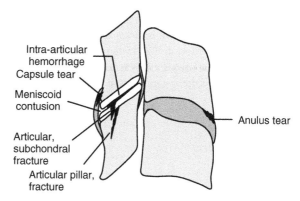

Figure 17.5 A sketch of the possible lesions of whiplash, as predicted by biomechanics studies.

neck pain or stiffness. In some cases the symptoms were of brief duration only immediately after impact,[14] but in others they lasted hours,[5] days,[5,15] or up to 2 weeks.[16] For fear of inducing more serious injury, laboratory studies have avoided collisions at speeds greater than 10 kph.

PATHOLOGY

Rare injuries which have been attributed to whiplash include disruption of the alar ligaments, prevertebral hematoma, perforation of the esophagus, tears of the sympathetic trunk, damage to the recurrent laryngeal nerve, spinal cord injury, periplymph fistula, thrombosis or traumatic aneurysms of the vertebral or internal carotid arteries, retinal angiopathy, and anterior spinal artery syndrome.[17,18] Fractures after whiplash are so uncommon as to be rare. Such fractures as have been attributed to whiplash have been reported only in case studies or small, descriptive series. These fractures may be difficult to detect by conventional investigations, and special attention needs to be paid to the possibility of their presence if they are to be detected. The majority involve the upper cervical spine, and include fractures of the odontoid process,[19,20] the laminae and articular processes of C2,[19,20,21] and the occipital condyles.[22] In one study of 283 patients with acute neck pain after whiplash, however, no fractures were found on plain radiography.[23] This result implies a prevalence of less than 1.3%. Another study, of 866 patients, found fractures in 26; which amounts to a prevalence of 3%.[24]

In the majority of patients, no lesion is evident on radiography. Modern imaging techniques do not provide the resolution necessary to detect the types of lesions predicted by the biomechanics studies. The lesions are not lethal, so post-mortem studies are difficult to conduct.[25] Surrogate data, however, are available that indicate what the lesions possibly might be.

Investigators in Sweden and in Australia examined the cervical spines of victims of fatal traffic accidents.[26,27,28,29] They censored what could be construed as the lethal injuries, such as suboccipital fractures, and focused on what comprised sublethal injuries as an index of what might occur in whiplash. Consistently and frequently they identified tears of the anterior anulus fibrosus, tears of the capsules of the zygapophysial joints, contusions of their meniscoids, intra-articular hemorrhage, subchondral fractures, and fractures of the articular pillars.

These injuries are consonant with what the biomechanics of whiplash predict could be the lesions of whiplash. None of the lesions, however, was evident on post-mortem radiography, which underscores the lack of resolution of radiography for lesions in capsular and ligamentous tissues, or for small fractures.

Additional, circumstantial evidence is available from two studies of cadavers subjected to whiplash impacts. One found injuries to the intervertebral discs in 90% of 21 cadavers, tears of the anterior longitudinal ligament in 80%, and tears of the zygapophysial joint capsules in 40%.[30] The other found tears in the anulus fibrosus, the anterior longitudinal ligament, and the zygapophysial joints of four cadavers tested.[31] Of the 12 lesions found on cryomicrotomy, only two were evident or suggested on plain radiography, and three on computed tomography.

IMPLICATIONS

Most importantly for clinical purposes, the biomechanics studies do not imply that every patient will sustain all or any of these lesions. It may be that many victims of whiplash escape any injury. Indeed, the epidemiological data suggest that the majority of victims suffer no substantive injury (Chapter 4). Any injury that they suffer is minor, for the majority recover.

Where the biomechanics evidence becomes relevant is in the interpretation of chronic neck pain after whiplash. In that context the biomechanics evidence serves two purposes.

For medicolegal purposes, the evidence dispels any notion that the neck cannot be injured during whiplash. The evidence clearly shows that abnormal motions occur, even in low-speed collisions, and that these motions can injure various components of the neck. At higher speeds of collision such as those encountered outside controlled laboratory conditions, the forces involved will be greater and must be more likely to cause injury.

For clinical purposes, the biomechanics evidence indicates what the possible injuries may be that cause symptoms. That information serves to guide investigations and treatment to the possible source of pain.

References

1. Bogduk N, Yoganandan N. Biomechanics of the cervical spine. Part 3. Minor injuries. Clin Biomech 2001; 16: 267–275.
2. Hammacher ER, van der Werken C. Acute neck sprain: 'whiplash' reappraised. Injury 1996; 27: 463–466.
3. Merskey H, Bogduk N (eds). Classification of Chronic Pain. IASP Press, Seattle, 1994: 107.
4. Bogduk N. The anatomy and pathophysiology of whiplash. Clin Biomech 1986; 1: 92–101.
5. McConnell WE, Howard RP, Guzman HM et al. Analysis of human test subject kinematic responses to low velocity rear end impacts. Proceedings of the 37th Stapp Car Crash Conference, San Antonio, TX, 1993: 21–30.
6. Panjabi MM, Pearson AM, Ito S, Ivancic PC, Wang JL. Cervical spine curvature during simulated whiplash. Clin Biomech 2004; 19: 1–9.
7. Pearson AM, Ivancic PC, Ito S, Panjabi MM. Facet joint kinematics and injury mechanisms during simulated whiplash. Spine 2004; 29: 390–397.
8. Kaneoka K, Ono K, Inami S, Hayashi K. Motion analysis of cervical vertebrae during whiplash loading. Spine 1999; 24: 763–770.
9. Grauer JN, Panjabi MM, Cholewicki J, Nibu K, Dvorak J. Whiplash produces an S-shaped curvature of the neck with hyperextension at lower levels. Spine 1997; 22: 2489–2494.
10. Cusick JF, Pintar FA, Yoganandan N. Whiplash syndrome: kinematic factors influencing pain patterns. Spine 2001; 26: 1252–1258.
11. Amevo B, Worth D, Bogduk N. Instantaneous axes of rotation of the typical cervical motion segments: a study in normal volunteers. Clin Biomech 1991; 6: 111–117.
12. Panjabi MM, Ito S, Pearson AM, Ivancic PC. Injury mechanisms of the cervical intervertebral disc during simulated whiplash. Spine 2004; 29: 1217–1225.
13. Panjabi MM, Cholewicki J, Nibu K, Grauer J, Vahldiek M. Capsular ligament stretches during in vitro whiplash simulations. J Spinal Dis 1998; 11: 227–232.
14. Szabo TJ, Welcher JB, Anderson RD et al. Human occupant kinematic response to low speed rear-end impacts. Proceedings of the Society for Automotive Engineers Conference, 1994: 630–642.
15. Matsushita T, Sato TB, Hirabayashi K, Fujimara S, Asazuma T. X-ray study of the human neck motion due to head inertia loading. Proceedings of the 38th Stapp Car Crash Conference, Fort Lauderdale, FL, 1994: 55–64.
16. Muhlbauer M, Eichberger A, Geigl BC, Steffan H. Analysis of kinematics and acceleration behaviour of the head and neck in experimental rear-impact collisions. Neuro-Orthopaedics 1999; 25: 1–17.
17. Barnsley L, Lord S, Bogduk N. Clinical review: whiplash injuries. Pain 1994; 58: 283–307.
18. Barnsley L, Lord SM, Bogduk N. The pathophysiology of whiplash. In: Malanga GA, Nadler SF. Whiplash. Hanley and Belfus, Philadelphia, 2002: 41–77.
19. Seletz E. Whiplash injuries: neurophysiological basis for pain and methods used for rehabilitation. JAMA 1958; 168: 1750–1755.
20. Signoret F, Feron JM, Bonfait H, Patel A. Fractured odontoid with fractured superior articular process of the axis. J Bone Joint Surg 1986; 68B: 182–184.
21. Craig JB, Hodgson BF. Superior facet fractures of the axis vertebra. Spine 1991; 16: 875–877.
22. Stroobants J, Fidler L, Storms JL, Klaes R, Dua G, van Hoye M. High cervical pain and impairment of skull mobility as the only symptoms of an occipital condyle fracture. J Neurosurg 1994; 81: 137–138.
23. Hoffman JR, Schriger DL, Mower W, Luo JS, Zucker M. Low-risk criteria for cervical-spine radiography in blunt trauma: a prospective study. Ann Emerg Med 1992; 21: 1454–1460.
24. Ovadia D, Steinberg EL, Nissan M, Dekel S. Whiplash injury: a retrospective study on patients seeking compensation. Injury 2002; 33: 569–573.
25. Bogduk N. Point of view. Cervical spine lesions after road traffic accidents: a systematic review. Spine 2002; 27: 1940–1941.
26. Jónsson H, Bring G, Rauschning W, Sahlstedt B. Hidden cervical spine injuries in traffic accident victims with skull fractures. J Spinal Disorders 1991; 4: 251–263.
27. Taylor JR, Twomey LT. Acute injuries to cervical joints: an autopsy study of neck sprain. Spine 1993; 9: 1115–1122.
28. Taylor JR, Taylor MM. Cervical spinal injuries: an autopsy study of 109 blunt injuries. J Musculoskelet Pain 1996; 4: 61–79.
29. Uhrenholdt L, Grunnet-Nilsson N, Hartvigsen K. Cervical spine lesions after road traffic accidents: a systematic review. Spine 2002; 27: 1934–1941.
30. Clemens HJ, Burow K. Experimental investigation on injury mechanisms of cervical spine at frontal and rear-frontal vehicle impacts. Proceedings of the 16th Stapp Car Crash Conference, Detroit, MI, 1972: 76–104.
31. Yoganandan N, Cusick JF, Pintar FA, Rao RD. Whiplash injury determination with conventional spine imaging and cryomicrotomy. Spine 2001; 26: 2443–2448.

Whiplash: mechanisms of symptoms

SYMPTOMS

Various symptoms have been attributed to whiplash injury (Table 18.1). Of these, neck pain and referred pain to the head or to the upper limb are the most prevalent and consistent. Indeed, pain is the defining clinical feature of whiplash, and is the only symptom readily attributed to an injury to the cervical spine. The other features that have variously been attributed to whiplash occur less frequently and variably in samples of patients.

REFERENCES

1. Maimaris C, Barnes MR, Allen MJ. "Whiplash injuries" of the neck: a retrospective study. Injury 1988; 19: 393–396.
2. Dvorak J, Valach L, Schmid ST. Cervical spine injuries in Switzerland. J Manual Med 1989; 4: 7–16.
3. Radanov BP, Sturzenegger M, Di Stefano G. Long-term outcome after whiplash injury: a 2-year follow-up considering features of injury mechanism and somatic, radiologic, and psychosocial findings. Medicine 1995; 74: 281–297.
4. Hildingsson C, Toolanen G. Outcome after soft tissue injury of the cervical spine: a prospective study of 93 car-accident victims. Acta Orthop Scand 1990; 61: 357–359.
5. Sturzenegger M, Di Stefano G, Radanov B, Schnidring A. Presenting symptoms and signs after whiplash injury: the influence of accident mechanisms. Neurology 1994; 44: 688–693.
6. Lord S, Barnsley L, Wallis BJ, Bogduk N. Chronic cervical zygapophysial joint pain after whiplash: a placebo-controlled prevalence study. Spine 1996; 21: 1737–1745.
7. Ovadia D, Steinberg EL, Nissan M, Dekel S. Whiplash injury: a retrospective study on patients seeking compensation. Injury 2002; 33: 569–573.

LESSER SYMPTOMS

Because the lesser symptoms of whiplash have attracted little specific study, their mechanisms have not been demonstrated. Nevertheless, various conjectures have been invoked to explain how these symptoms might be generated.[1,2] Without suggesting that these explanations have been verified, they are outlined below.

Table 18.1 The incidence of various symptoms in selected studies of patients with whiplash

Symptom	Proportion of patients (%) reporting symptoms						
	Acute				*Chronic*		
	A	*B*	*C*	*D*	*E*	*F*	*G*
Pain							
—Neck pain	89	90	92	88	74	100	95
—Headache	26		57	54	33	88	20
—Shoulder pain	37	80	49	40			61
Other							
—Paresthesia		50	15		45	68	
—Weakness						68	
—Dizziness		62	15	23		53	12
—Visual problems				9	2	42	14
—Tinnitus		30	4	4	14		
—Cognitive impairment		26				71	
—Back pain		42	39		42		
Sample size	102	320	117	93	43	68	866

A: Maimaris et al.[1] *B:* Dvorak et al.[2] *C:* Radanov et al.[3] *D:* Hildingsson and Toolanen[4]. *E:* Sturzenegger et al.[5] *F:* Lord et al.[6] *G:* Ovadia et al.[7]

PARESTHESIA

Not all studies of whiplash patients list paresthesia as a symptom. This might be because different studies have used different selection criteria. According to the Quebec Task Force,[3] patients who lack neurological symptoms would be classified as whiplash-associated disorder grade I or II (WAD I or II). Those with neurological symptoms constitute WAD III.

Paresthesia is a neurological symptom typical of cervical radiculopathy so it could be a symptom of patients with WAD III. Its presence invites investigation for radiculopathy.

However, not all patients with paresthesia have other evidence of radiculopathy, such as dermatomal numbness, myotomal weakness, or loss of reflexes. Furthermore, their paresthesia may not be dermatomal in distribution. This irregularity does not constitute evidence that the symptom is not genuine. Explanations other than radiculopathy apply.

It is conceivable and feasible that tightened scalene muscles may narrow the thoracic outlet and compress the roots of the brachial plexus. That compression would result in paresthesia in a so-called glove distribution, but would be consistent with the C6, C7, and C8 roots of the plexus all being compressed. This explanation would be particularly apposite when the paresthesia is intermittent and associated with exacerbations of pain.

The intermittent nature of the symptom indicates absence of a fixed lesion, such as a disc protrusion or foraminal stenosis, and is more consistent with a fluctuating abnormality such as muscle tightness in response to pain.

WEAKNESS

Weakness in a myotomal distribution implies radiculopathy, but patients with whiplash more often complain of a global weakness. This irregularity is not a sign that the complaint is not genuine.

Physiological studies have shown that patients experience a subjective sensation of weakness when the affected body part is subjected to pain.[4,5] Nociceptive input inhibits the motor neuron pools of those muscles that move the painful part. The muscles are not weak in the sense that they are denervated. Rather, the patient needs to exert a greater upper motor neuron drive in order to overcome the segmental inhibition.

In the context of weakness associated with neck pain, the model would be that any motor effort that stresses the cervical spine aggravates the neck pain, which inhibits the effort. In that regard, movements that invoke the levator scapulae and rhomboid muscles, directly or indirectly, will exert compression loads on the neck and threaten to aggravate neck pain. These movements will, therefore, appear subjectively weak.

This relationship will be particularly evident if patients are examined in an upright position, for in that position any muscle testing will recruit muscles of the scapula to stabilize the shoulder girdle as effort is increased. One way of avoiding this confounding effect is to examine the patient supine and with the shoulder girdle braced. Doing so mechanically isolates the distal upper limb from the shoulder girdle, and avoids transmission of reaction forces into the neck. Under those conditions, the strength of the muscles of the hand, wrist, and elbow can be tested without aggravating the neck pain.

DIZZINESS

Dizziness is a perplexing problem in patients with whiplash. Two types of explanation can be invoked.

One model is that dizziness implies some sort of damage to the balance organs of the inner ear. For this reason, some investigators have pursued entities such as perilymph fistulas in patients with whiplash injuries.[6,7] The difficulties in studying the inner ear, however, have been a barrier to the promotion of this model.

Another model is that dizziness is a feature of damage to tonic neck reflexes, for which reason it has been called cervical vertigo. The grounds for this model lie in multiple animal experiments[8,9] and clinical experimental studies[10,11] in which disturbances of balance have been induced by noxious stimulation of the posterior neck muscles, or by anesthetizing nerves to those muscles. Indeed, blocking upper cervical nerves regularly induces a form of ataxia. It is not vertigo, for it does not involve a spinning sensation. Rather, it is a sense of unsteadiness, like being drunk. That quality of sensation would be consistent with spinovestibular pathways being affected.

However, there are no objective tests whereby this model can be tested directly. There are no means by which excess or deficient spinovestibular activity can be detected. But indirect evidence is available. Patients with whiplash injuries have normal pursuit performance of their eyes, if head movements are not required. But once the pursuit requires rotation of the head by the neck, the pursuit becomes demonstrably abnormal. This abnormality implies a disturbance in spinovestibular control of optokinetic pursuit.

It is not evident that dizziness due to neck injury is caused by damage to cervical proprioreceptors. It seems more likely that is secondary to disturbed function of the cervical muscles, which in turn is secondary to the pain experienced by the patient.

VISUAL PROBLEMS

The visual problems reported by patients with whiplash injuries are poorly defined in the literature,

even though they are commonly reported. Patients who report the symptom have difficulty describing it. It is not a visual loss but more like difficulty focusing.

Explanations of this phenomenon center around the spinociliary reflex. Classically, the spinociliary reflex is a test of the integrity of the cervical sympathetic nerves. If the nerves are intact, scratching the skin of the neck elicits dilation of the ipsilateral pupil of the eye. Absence of dilation implies interruption of the dilation pathway.

In principle, therefore, the spinociliary reflex is a link between cervical nociception and dilation of the pupil. It is feasible, therefore, that patients with neck pain may have increased dilator tone, driven by this reflex. To overcome that tone, patients need to increase the drive for the constriction required to focus on near objects. A side-effect of that increased drive would be increased accommodation. If this effect is unilateral, the accommodation in each eye would be asymmetrical, resulting in a confusing sensation of inappropriate focus, perceived as blurred vision.

TINNITUS

Tinnitus is the most inexplicable symptom of whiplash. Beyond invoking some sort of injury to the inner ear, commentators have not been able to produce an attractive explanation.

COGNITIVE IMPAIRMENT

Some investigators have sought to attribute the cognitive impairment of whiplash to brain damage. They have investigated their patients with electroencephalography, brain scans, and PET scans. The resultant evidence has not been conclusive.

Rather than a direct result of whiplash injury, it is more likely that disturbances in memory or concentration are secondary to persistent pain or to the side-effects of drugs used to treat the pain.[2]

BACK PAIN

Back pain is commonly reported by patients with whiplash (Table 18.1), but this symptom has not been explicitly studied. It is not known if back pain is attributable to whiplash, or if its prevalence represents no more than the endemic prevalence of back pain in the community. One explanation is that patients may injure their back if and when their seat back collapses during a rear-end collision. Beyond speculation, this mechanism of injury has not been explored.

REFERENCES

1. Barnsley L, Lord S, Bogduk N. Clinical review: whiplash injuries. Pain 1994; 58: 283–307.

2. Barnsley L, Lord SM, Bogduk N. The pathophysiology of whiplash. In: Malanga GA, Nadler SF. Whiplash. Hanley and Belfus, Philadelphia, 2002: 41–77.

3. Spitzer WO, Skovron ML, Salmi LR et al. Scientific monograph of the Quebec task force on whiplash-associated disorders: redefining "whiplash" and its management. Spine 1995; 20: 1S–73S.

4. Gandevia SC, McCloskey DI. Sensations of heaviness. Brain 1977; 100: 345–354.

5. Aniss AM, Gandevia SC, Milne RJ. Changes in perceived heaviness and motor commands produced by cutaneous reflexes in man. J Physiol 1988; 397: 113–126.

6. Grimm RJ, Hemenway WG, Lebray PR. The perilymph fistula syndrome defined in mild head trauma. Acta Otolaryngol 1989; 464(Suppl.): 1–40.

7. Chester JB. Whiplash, postural control, and the inner ear. Spine 1991; 16: 716–720.

8. Igarashi M, Alford BR, Watanabe T, Maxian PM. Role of neck proprioceptors in the maintenance of dynamic body equilibrium in the squirrel monkey. Laryngoscope 1969; 79: 1713–1727.

9. Igarashi M, Miyata H, Alford BR, Wright WK. Nystagmus after experimental cervical lesions. Laryngoscope 1972; 82: 1609–1621.

10. Biemond A, de Jong JMBV. On cervical nystagmus and related disorders. Brain 1969; 92: 437–458.

11. de Jong PTVM, de Jong JMBV, Cohen B, Jongkees LBW. Ataxia and nystagmus caused by injection of local anaesthetic in the neck. Ann Neurol 1977; 1: 240–246.

PAIN

The available biomechanics and pathology evidence indicates that the neck can be injured by whiplash (Chapter 17). The possible lesions include sprains of the anterior anulus fibrosus and tears and impaction injuries of the zygapophysial joints. Each of these lesions constitutes a possible basis for pain. It should not be contentious, therefore, that pain would be a symptom of whiplash.

The primary site of pain would be in the cervical spine, but if severe enough, that pain could be referred. From upper cervical segments it could be referred to the head. From lower cervical segments it could be referred to the shoulder girdle or to the anterior chest wall (Chapter 2). It is not just possible but is to be expected that neck pain, headache, and shoulder pain would be symptoms of whiplash injury.

IMPLICATIONS

For the major symptoms of whiplash, namely neck pain and pain referred to the head or to the shoulder region, there is sufficient circumstantial evidence to provide an explanation. The biomechanics evidence indicates that various structures can be injured during whiplash, and the predicted lesions have been corroborated by post-mortem studies (Chapter 17). So, pain should be an acceptable symptom after whiplash. The challenge for practitioners is only to identify the source of pain in individual patients (Chapter 13).

For the lesser symptoms of whiplash, evidence is lacking. However, for medicolegal purposes it is not true that these symptoms cannot be explained. Explanations have been provided in the literature. The statement that is true is that there is no evidence that these explanations are correct. The complementary statement is that there is no evidence that the symptoms are not valid or that they cannot possibly be due to whiplash.

Furthermore, there are good reasons why the evidence is lacking. Several of the lesser symptoms involve body systems that are difficult to study. There are no means, at present, by which vestibular, acoustic and visual systems can be studied directly in vivo, to test conjectural mechanisms or to establish others. As well, these symptoms are not seriously debilitating, and have not been attractive topics for research.

A conspicuous feature of the lesser symptoms apart from tinnitus is that they can all be explained in terms of a secondary response to pain. The ultimate test of that relationship is that they should resolve spontaneously if pain is relieved. However, that test has not been applied because so few treatments, when used for whiplash, have been shown to stop pain completely. Meanwhile, no studies have sought to relieve any of the lesser symptoms directly. *The treatment of whiplash amounts to the treatment of neck pain.*

5 Cervicogenic headache

Cervicogenic headache: overview

The entity known as cervicogenic headache is besieged with conflict. At least four craft groups have contributed not only to the recognition of this entity but also to the tensions concerning it (Figure 19.1).

Manual therapists have long contended that disorders of the cervical spine can cause a certain form of headache. Indeed, they were among the earliest contributors to the contemporary debate about this issue.[1] The distinction proffered by manual therapists is that purportedly these headaches can be diagnosed by detecting, by manual examination, abnormalities in the joints of the cervical spine that are responsible for the pain.

Some headache specialists promoted cervicogenic headache as a distinctive entity that could be diagnosed on the basis of a particular set of conventional clinical features.[2,3] Those features did not involve abnormalities of joints detected by manual examination. Rather, they involved the site of pain, its quality, and certain gross features suggestive of a cervical source of pain, such as restricted range of motion, provocation of headache by neck movements, and tenderness in the neck.

Pain specialists took a different approach. Accustomed to diagnosing spinal pain with diagnostic blocks or other needle procedures, they defined cervicogenic headache in a like manner. To them the critical diagnostic criterion was relief of pain following anesthetization of a cervical structure or its nerve supply.[4,5,6,7] Other clinical features were not required for the diagnosis.

Overseeing this evolution and conflict of concepts have been neurologists with a special interest in headaches. Not all have embraced the concept of cervicogenic headache. Some have been critical of it, basing their criticism on lack of a demonstrable pathology for this condition.[8]

Each of these participants has made valuable, positive contributions to the evolution of the concept but, as outlined in Chapters 22, 23, and 24, they have also failed in several respects to bring those contributions to fruition. The deficiencies provide footholds for opponents to maintain criticism of the concept.

Ironically, however, if the literature is reviewed thoroughly it transpires that cervicogenic headaches are one the best understood forms of headache, and one of the few common headaches that can be diagnosed objectively. The controversies that surround this entity are more sociological, ideological,

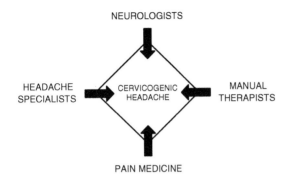

Figure 19.1 Groups that have contributed both to the development of the concept of cervicogenic headache and to its controversies.

and political than scientific. The problems can be understood by reviewing the anatomical basis of the concept, its history, problems of diagnosis, and deficiencies of treatment.

REFERENCES

1. Bogduk N, Corrigan B, Kelly P, Schneider G, Farr R. Cervical headache. Med J Aust 1985; 143: 202–207.
2. Fredriksen TA, Hovdal H, Sjaastad O. "Cervicogenic headache": clinical manifestation. Cephalalgia 1987; 7: 147–160.
3. Sjaastad O, Fredriksen TA, Pfaffenrath V. Cervicogenic headache: diagnostic criteria. Headache 1990; 30: 725–726.
4. Bogduk N. Headaches and the cervical spine. An editorial. Cephalalgia 1984; 4: 7–8.
5. Bogduk N, Marsland A. On the concept of third occipital headache. J Neurol Neurosurg Psychiat 1986; 49: 775–780.
6. Rothbart P: Cervicogenic headache. Headache 1996; 36: 516.
7. Bogduk N. Headache and the neck. In: Goadsby PJ, Silberstein SD (eds). Headache. Butterworth-Heinemann, Boston, 1997: 369–381.
8. Gobel H, Edmeads JG. Disorders of the skull and cervical spine. In: Olesen J, Tfelt-Hansen P, Welch KMA (eds). The Headaches, 2nd edn. Lippincott Williams and Wilkins, Philadelphia, 2000: 891–898.

Cervicogenic headache: an abridged summary

This chapter provides a concise summary of the information concerning cervicogenic headaches that is likely to be of interest, but, more importantly, of use to practitioners unfamiliar with this entity. For readers interested in a fuller exposition of the data and evidence, or for those interested in a defense of the conclusions provided in this chapter, Chapters 21, 22, 23, and 24 cover the anatomical basis, diagnosis, and treatment of cervicogenic headaches in extended detail.

DEFINITION

Cervicogenic headache is pain that is perceived in the head but whose source is actually in the cervical spine or which is innervated by cervical nerves. It amounts to a particular form of cervical referred pain.[1,2,3]

MECHANISM

Sensory axons in the C1, 2, and 3 spinal nerves converge on dorsal horn neurons that also receive trigeminal afferents, largely from the ophthalmic division. This convergence allows pain mediated by the C1, 2, or 3 nerves to be perceived in regions innervated by the trigeminal nerve.[1,2,3]

CLINICAL FEATURES

There are no distinctive clinical features of cervicogenic headache. It is manifest essentially, if not exclusively, by pain in the occipital, parietal, frontal, or orbital regions of the head, or in some combination of these regions.

DIAGNOSTIC CRITERIA

The International Headache Society[4] has stipulated the following diagnostic criteria for cervicogenic headache:

A. Pain referred from a source in the neck and perceived in one or more regions of the head and/or face, fulfilling criteria C and D.

B. Clinical, laboratory and/or imaging evidence of a disorder or lesion within the cervical spine or soft tissues of the neck known to be, or generally accepted as, a valid cause of headache.[a]

C. Evidence that the pain can be attributed to the neck disorder or lesion based on at least one of the following:

1. demonstration of clinical signs that implicate a source of pain in the neck[b]
2. abolition of headache following diagnostic blockade of a cervical structure or its nerve supply using placebo or other adequate controls.[c]

The footnotes to these criteria specify that:

[a.] Tumors, fractures, infections and rheumatoid arthritis of the upper cervical spine have not been validated formally as causes of headache, but are nevertheless accepted as valid causes when demonstrated to be so in individual cases. Cervical spondylosis and osteochondritis are NOT accepted as valid causes fulfilling criterion B. When myofascial tender spots are evident, the headache should be coded under 2. *Tension-type headache.*

[b.] Clinical signs acceptable for criterion C1 must have demonstrated reliability and validity. The future task is the identification of such reliable and valid operational tests. Clinical features such as neck pain, focal neck tenderness, history of neck trauma, mechanical exacerbation of pain, unilaterality, coexisting shoulder pain, reduced range of motion in the neck, nuchal onset, nausea, vomiting, photophobia, etc. are not unique to cervicogenic headache. These may be features of cervicogenic headache, but they do not define relationship between the disorder and the source of the headache.

[c.] Abolition of headache means complete relief of headache, indicated by a score of zero on a visual analogue scale (VAS). Nevertheless, acceptable as fulfilling criterion C2 is $\geq$ 90% reduction in pain to a level of < 5 on a 100-point scale.

CAUSES

The possible and putative causes of cervicogenic headache can be divided into detectable but rare conditions and common conditions, some of which are detectable but others of which are contentious (Table 20.1). There are also causes that have been refuted.

Rare causes

The differential diagnosis of cervicogenic headache includes *aneurysms* of the vertebral artery and of the internal carotid artery, as well as *tumors* and *infections* of the posterior cranial fossa.[2,3] These conditions would be suspected on the basis of their distinctive history and associated clinical features. The diagnosis would be confirmed by angiography, lumbar puncture, or magnetic resonance imaging.

Table 20.1 The causes of cervicogenic headache

	Detectable	*Putative*
Rare	Aneurysms Tumors and infections of the posterior cranial fossa Neck tongue syndrome C2 neuralgia	
Common	Third occipital headache Lateral atlanto-axial joint pain	Median atlanto-axial joint pain Atlanto-occipital joint pain C2–3 intervertebral disc pain

Neck tongue syndrome is a distinctive entity defined by the sudden onset of occipital headache upon turning of the head, associated with a sense of numbness in the ipsilateral half of the tongue.[2,3] It is caused by subluxation of the lateral atlanto-axial joint and stretching the C2 spinal nerve behind the joint.

C2 neuralgia is characterized by paroxysmal, lancinating pain in the occiput. It is caused by irritation of the C2 spinal nerve by periarticular fibrosis, nerve tumors, or vascular malformations. The diagnosis is essentially based on the distinctive character of the pain, but can be confirmed anesthetizing the C2 spinal nerve.[2,3]

Common causes

Third occipital headache is pain arising from the C2–3 zygapophysial joint and mediated by the third occipital nerve, which innervates this joint. It is the best studied of all causes of cervicogenic headache.[2,3] It accounts for 53% of patients with headache after whiplash. This form of headache is diagnosed by blocking the third occipital nerve.

The *lateral atlanto-axial joint* (C1–2) is emerging as a possible, and common, source of cervicogenic headache, but the available literature falls short of being definitive.[2,3] Pain from this joint can be diagnosed by anesthetizing the C1–2 joint.

Putative causes

Osteoarthrosis, or some other disorder, of the other upper cervical joints is a possible basis for cervicogenic headache.[2,3] These joints include the median atlanto-axial joint and the atlanto-occipital joints. Atlanto-occipital joint pain can be diagnosed by blocking the joint, but no studies have yet reported the yield from such blocks. No technique has been developed for diagnosing pain from the median atlanto-axial joint. It is incriminated, but only weakly, by finding arthritic changes on CT scans of this joint.

Refuted causes

Occipital neuralgia is a dated and contentious diagnostic label. There are no agreed or consistent diagnostic criteria.[2,3] Patients who have attracted this label in the past probably had C2 neuralgia or pain from the upper cervical joints.

Barré syndrome, or *migraine cervicale*, is another dated entity. It used to be believed that headache could be caused by irritation of the sympathetic nerves that accompany the vertebral artery. Physiological studies have refuted this mechanism.[2,3] Meanwhile no clinical studies have validated the entity.[2,3]

Trigger points have long been held to be a cause of headache, but no studies have ever vindicated this entity. The diagnostic criteria for trigger points in the upper cervical spine lack both reliability and validity.[2,3] Trigger points cannot be distinguished clinically from underlying tender joints.[2,3]

DIAGNOSIS

The diagnostic criteria of the International Headache Society[4] are rigorous and demanding. They require reliable and valid tests if the diagnosis is to be made clinically, but no such tests have yet been established. Such tests as have been used to diagnose cervicogenic headache in the past lack validity, and most lack reliability.[5]

Only two definitive means of making a diagnosis are currently available. The serious and rare causes can be detected by medical imaging for aneurysms, tumors, or infection. The common causes can be diagnosed by anesthetizing the upper cervical joint suspected of being the source of pain.

Diagnostic blocks, however, require special skills and special facilities, for they must be performed under fluoroscopic guidance. For practitioners to make the diagnosis they need to be able to refer their patients to a colleague experienced in performing these blocks accurately.

A less rigorous, but pragmatic, alternative approach can be used in the first instance. A diagnosis of *possible* cervicogenic headache can be applied if the headache is unilateral headache, and the pain appears to start in the neck.[5] This diagnosis is promoted to *probable* cervicogenic headache if the patient also has three additional features suggestive of a cervical source of pain, such as pain triggered by neck movements, sustained awkward posture, or by external pressure on the posterior neck or occipital region; reduced range of motion of the neck; ipsilateral neck, shoulder or arm pain; or a recent history of neck trauma.[5]

For practical purposes, a diagnosis of probable cervicogenic headache allows practitioners to undertake a trial of suitable treatment. The pursuit of a definitive diagnosis, using diagnostic blocks, can then be reserved for patients who do not respond to treatment.

TREATMENT

No drugs have been shown to be effective for cervicogenic headache.[6] Indeed, conventional care by a general practitioner, centered on analgesics, has been shown to be less effective than other measures.[7]

The only forms of treatment that have been validated for *probable* cervicogenic headache are manual therapy, exercises, or manual therapy combined with exercises.[7] Each is similarly effective. Practitioners wishing to avail their patients of these interventions could enlist the services of a physical therapist or a medical colleague skilled in these interventions.

For patients with third occipital headache, in whom the diagnosis has been established by controlled diagnostic blocks, two specific interventions are available. Intra-articular injections of steroids, into the C2–3 zygapophysial joint, can be effective in a modest proportion of patients.[5] Otherwise, the only means known to relieve third occipital headache completely is radiofrequency neurotomy.

Radiofrequency neurotomy involves coagulating the third occipital nerve with an electrode inserted percutaneously under fluoroscopic guidance.[5] It provides complete relief of pain in 86% of patients. If pain recurs, relief can be reinstated by repeating the procedure.

Cervicogenic headache stemming from the C2–3 intervertebral disc can be treated by arthrodesis of the disc.[8] There are no proven treatments for any other form of cervicogenic headache.

References

1. Bogduk N. Mechanisms and pain patterns of the upper cervical spine. In: Vernon H (ed). The Cranio-Cervical Syndrome: Mechanisms, Assessment and Treatment. Butterworth Heinemann, Oxford, 2001: 110–116.
2. Bogduk N. The neck and headaches. Neurol Clin N Am 2004; 22: 151–171.
3. Bogduk N. Headache and the neck. In: Goadsby PJ, Silberstein SD (eds). Headache. Butterworth-Heinemann, Boston, 1997: 369–381.
4. International Headache Society. The International Classification of Headache Disorders, 2nd edn. Cephalalgia 2004; 24(Suppl. 1): 115–116.
5. Bogduk N. Current review. Distinguishing primary headache disorders from cervicogenic headache: clinical and therapeutic implications. Headache Currents 2005; 2: 27–36.
6. Bogduk N. Cervicogenic headache. In: Diener HC (ed). Drug Treatment of Migraine and Other Headaches. Monographs in Clinical Neuroscience, vol. 17. Karger, Basel, 2000: 357–362.
7. Jull G, Trott P, Potter H et al. A randomized controlled trial of exercise and manipulative therapy for cervicogenic headache. Spine 2002; 27: 1835–1843.
8. Schofferman J, Garges K, Goldthwaite N, Koestler M, Libby E. Upper cervical anterior diskectomy and fusion improves discogenic cervical headaches. Spine 2002; 27: 2240–2244.

Cervicogenic headache: anatomical basis

KEY POINTS

- The mechanism of cervicogenic headache is convergence between cervical and trigeminal afferents in the trigeminocervical nucleus.

- Convergence has been demonstrated in experimental studies on laboratory animals.

- Referral of pain to the head from cervical structures has been demonstrated in normal volunteers.

- The possible sources of cervicogenic headache are the joints, ligaments, muscles, dura, and arteries innervated by the upper three cervical nerves (C1,2,3).

- Anesthetizing upper cervical joints relieves headache in certain patients.

By definition, cervicogenic headache is pain in the head whose source lies somewhere in the cervical spine. Technically, therefore, cervicogenic headache constitutes a particular form of referred pain from the cervical spine. That definition implies an anatomical and physiological connection between the nerves of the cervical spine and the mechanisms of headache.

NEUROANATOMY

The pars caudalis of the spinal nucleus of the trigeminal nerve is continuous longitudinally with the outer laminae (laminae I to V) of the dorsal horns of the upper three to four segments of the cervical spinal cord.[1–7] Collectively, this column of gray matter constitutes the trigeminocervical nucleus. This nucleus, however, is not defined by any distinctive cytoarchitecture or by any intrinsic boundaries. Rather, it is defined by its afferents. The nucleus receives afferents from the trigeminal nerve and from the upper three cervical spinal nerves[3] (Figure 21.1). Within the nucleus, second-order neurons receive

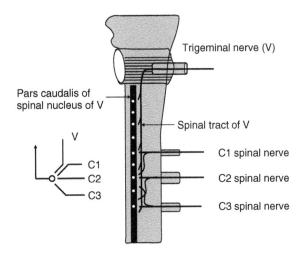

Figure 21.1 A sketch of the location in the brainstem of the trigeminocervical nucleus and the manner in which it receives overlapping afferents from the trigeminal nerve and the C1,2,3 spinal nerves. The inset shows the manner of convergence between these afferents within the nucleus.

afferents both from the trigeminal nerve and from the upper three cervical spinal nerves. This convergence provides for various patterns of referred pain.

Convergence between cervical spinal afferents from the vertebral column and cervical afferents from the occiput provides for cervical–cervical referral of pain. Thereby, pain from upper cervical spinal structures

may be perceived in regions of the head innervated by cervical nerves, such as the external occiput or the posterior cranial fossa. Convergence between cervical afferents and trigeminal afferents provides for cervical-trigeminal referral. Thereby, pain from upper cervical spinal structures can be perceived in the frontal region of the head, or the orbit, or the parietal region.

PERIPHERAL ANATOMY

The possible sources of cervical spinal pain that might be referred to the head are dictated by the distribution of the upper three cervical spinal nerves. Through their various branches these nerves innervate: the joints and ligaments of the median atlanto-axial joint,[8] the atlanto-occipital[9] and lateral atlanto-axial joints,[9,10] the C2–3 zygapophysial joint,[11] the suboccipital and upper posterior neck muscles,[11] the upper prevertebral muscles,[12] the spinal dura mater and the dura mater of the posterior cranial fossa,[8] the vertebral artery,[13,14,15] the C2–3 intervertebral disc,[16,17] and the trapezius and sternocleidomastoid muscles.[12] Collectively, these structures constitute the possible sources of headache referred from the cervical spine (Table 21.1).

HUMAN EXPERIMENTAL EVIDENCE

Studies in human volunteers have demonstrated the patterns of referred pain that can occur from cervical structures to the head. Electrical stimulation of the dorsal rootlets of C1 produces frontal headache.[18]

Table 21.1 The possible sources of cervicogenic headache, listed according to innervation and type of structure

| Structure | *Innervation* | | |
	C1	**C2**	**C3**
Joints	Median atlanto-axial		
	Atlanto-occipital	Lateral atlanto-axial	C2–3 zygapophysial
			C2–3 disc
Ligaments	Transverse atlanto-axial and alar; membrana tectoria		
Muscles	Prevertebral; sternocleidomastoid, trapezius		
	Suboccipital	Semispinalis, splenius	
			Multifidus; semispinalis
Dura	Upper spinal cord; posterior cranial fossa		
Arteries	Vertebral; internal carotid		

Noxious stimulation of the greater occipital nerve produces headache in the ipsilateral, frontal and parietal regions.[19] Noxious stimulation of the suboccipital muscles of the neck produces pain in the forehead.[20-23] Noxious stimulation of the C2–3 intervertebral disc, but not lower discs, produces pain in the occipital region.[24,25] Distending the C2–3 zygapophysial joint with injections of contrast medium produces pain in the occipital region,[26] as does distending the lateral atlanto-axial joint or the atlanto-occipital joint.[27] In normal volunteers, all segments from the occiput to C4–5 are capable of producing referred pain to the occiput. Referral to the forehead and orbital regions more commonly occurs from the uppermost segments: C1 and C2.[21]

Complementary studies in patients with headache have shown that headache can be relieved by anesthetizing cervical structures. Anesthetizing the C2–3 zygapophysial joint[28,29,30] or the lateral atlanto-axial joint[31-34] relieves frontal and occipital headache in some patients. Systematic studies have shown that when headache is the dominant symptom the source is most commonly the C2–3 zygapophysial joint, and occasionally the joint at C3–4.[35] In patients with predominantly neck pain but in whom headache is also a feature but not the dominant complaint, zygapophysial joints as low as C5–6 can be the source of pain.[35]

LABORATORY EVIDENCE

Physiological studies, using a cat model, have demonstrated that various sites in the spinal cord at the C1–2 level respond to electrical stimulation of either the trigeminal nerve or the roots of the C1 or C2 spinal nerve.[36] More specifically, studies have shown that neurons in the lateral cervical nucleus respond to electrical stimulation of either the superior sagittal sinus or the greater occipital nerve.[37]

Two complementary studies,[38,39] in the rat, found neurons in the C2 spinal cord that received convergent input from both trigeminal and cervical afferents. Aδ and C fibers of these afferents converge on wide dynamic range neurons and nociceptive specific neurons located in laminae V and VI, and laminae I and II, of the dorsal horn at C2. The trigeminal afferents were stimulated at the dura mater of the parietal bone, but had receptive fields that extended to the cutaneous territories predominantly of the ophthalmic, but also the maxillary and mandibular divisions of the trigeminal nerve. The cervical afferents were stimulated in the greater occipital nerve, but had receptive fields both in the cutaneous territory of this nerve and in the muscles that it innervates.

Electrical or chemical stimulation of trigeminal afferents sensitizes the central neurons and increases their responses to cervical stimulation.[38,39] Reciprocally, electrical or chemical stimulation of cervical afferents sensitizes the neurons to trigeminal input. Thus, either trigeminal or cervical stimulation can produce central sensitization of the trigeminocervical nucleus.

These observations underscore the reciprocal nature of cervical-trigeminal interactions. Not only can cervical nociception facilitate trigeminal sensation, trigeminal nociception facilitates cervical perception. Consequently, the neurophysiological data support not only the referral of cervical pain to the head, but also the generation of cervical features in patients with trigeminal sources of headache. Proponents of a cervical source of headaches, therefore, need to be alert to the possibility that signs, which they infer indicate a cervical origin for pain, may instead be secondary phenomena of trigeminal origin. In experimental animals, stimulation of the dura mater increases electromyographic activity in suboccipital paraspinal muscles.[40] Migraine patients can complain of neck discomfort during the premonitory phase[41] or during their attacks;[42] and they can exhibit hypersensitivity and increased electromyographic activity in their neck muscles.[43,44,45]

References

1. Humphrey T. The spinal tract of the trigeminal nerve in human embryos between 71/2 and 81/2 weeks of menstrual age and its relation to early fetal behaviour. J Comp Neurol 1952; 97: 143–209.

2. Torvik A. Afferent connections to the sensory trigeminal nuclei, the nucleus of the solitary tract and adjacent structures. J Comp Neurol 1956; 106: 51–141.

3. Kerr FWL. Structural relation of the trigeminal spinal tract to upper cervical roots and the solitary nucleus in the cat. Exp Neurol 1961; 4: 134–148.

4. Taren JA, Kahn EA. Anatomic pathways related to pain in face and neck. J Neurosurg 1962; 19: 116–121.

5. Goadsby PJ, Hoskin KL. The distribution of trigeminovascular afferents in the nonhuman primate brain Macaca nemestrina: a c-fos immunocytochemical study. J Anat 1997; 190: 367–375.

6. Kaube H, Keay KA, Hoskin KL, Bandler R, Goadsby PJ. Expression of c-fos-like immunoreactivity in the caudal medulla and upper cervical spinal cord following stimulation of the superior sagittal sinus in the cat. Brain Res 1993; 629: 95–102.

7. Strassman AM, Potrevbic S, Maciewicz RJ. Anatomical properties of brainstem trigeminal neurons that respond to electrical stimulation of dural blood vessels. J Comp Neurol 1994; 346: 349–365.

8. Kimmel DL. Innervation of the spinal dura mater and dura mater of the posterior cranial fossa. Neurology 1960; 10: 800–809.

9. Lazorthes G, Gaubert J. L'innervation des articulations interapophysaire vertebrales. Comptes Rendues de l'Association des Anatomistes 1956: 488–494.

10. Bogduk N. Local anaesthetic blocks of the second cervical ganglion: a technique with application in occipital headache. Cephalalgia 1981; 1: 41–50.

11. Bogduk N. The clinical anatomy of the cervical dorsal rami. Spine 1982; 7: 319–330.

12. Williams PL, Warwick R, Dyson M, Bannister LH (eds). Gray's Anatomy, 37th edn. Churchill Livingstone, Edinburgh, 1989.

13. Hovelacque A. Anatomie des Nerfs Craniens et Rachidiens et du Système Grand Sympathique. Doin, Paris, 1927.

14. Bogduk N, Lambert G, Duckworth JW. The anatomy and physiology of the vertebral nerve in relation to cervical migraine. Cephalalgia 1981; 1: 1–14.

15. Kimmel DL. The cervical sympathetic rami and the vertebral plexus in the human foetus. J Comp Neurol 1959; 112: 141–161.

16. Bogduk N, Windsor M, Inglis A. The innervation of the cervical intervertebral discs. Spine 1989; 13: 2–8.

17. Mendel T, Wink CS, Zimny ML. Neural elements in human cervical intervertebral discs. Spine 1992; 17: 132–135.

18. Kerr FWL. A mechanism to account for frontal headache in cases of posterior fossa tumors. J Neurosurg 1962; 18: 605–609.

19. Piovesan EJ, Kowacs PA, Tatsui CE, Lange MC, Ribas LC, Werneck LC. Referred pain after painful stimulation of the greater occipital nerve in humans: evidence of convergence of cervical afferents on trigeminal nuclei. Cephalalgia 2001; 21: 107–109.

20. Cyriax J. Rheumatic headache. Brit Med J 1938; 2: 1367–1368.

21. Campbell DG, Parsons CM. Referred head pain and its concomitants. J Nerv Ment Dis 1944; 99: 544–551.

22. Feinstein B, Langton JBK, Jameson RM, Schiller F. Experiments on referred pain from deep somatic tissues. J Bone Joint Surg 1954; 36A: 981–997.

23. Wolff HG. Headache and Other Head Pain, 2nd edn. Oxford University Press, New York, 1963: 582–616.

24. Schellhas KP, Smith MD, Gundry CR, Pollei SR. Cervical discogenic pain: prospective correlation of magnetic resonance imaging and discography in asymptomatic subjects and pain sufferers. Spine 1996, 21: 300–312.

25. Grubb SA, Kelly CK. Cervical discography: clinical implications from 12 years of experience. Spine 2000, 25: 1382–1389.

26. Dwyer A, Aprill C, Bogduk N. Cervical zygapophysial joint pain patterns I: a study in normal volunteers. Spine 1990; 15: 453–457.

27. Dreyfuss P, Michaelsen M, Fletcher D. Atlanto-occipital and lateral atlanto-axial joint pain patterns. Spine 1994; 19: 1125–1131.

28. Bogduk N, Marsland A. On the concept of third occipital headache. J Neurol Neurosurg Psychiatry 1986; 49: 775–780.

29. Bogduk N, Marsland A. The cervical zygapophysial joints as a source of neck pain. Spine 1988; 13: 610–617.

30. Lord S, Barnsley L, Wallis B, Bogduk N. Third occipital headache: a prevalence study. J Neurol Neurosurg Psychiatry 1994; 57: 1187–1190.

31. Ehni G, Benner B. Occipital neuralgia and the C1-2 arthrosis syndrome. J Neurosurg 1984; 61: 961–965.

32. McCormick CC. Arthrography of the atlanto-axial (C1–C2) joints: technique and results. J Intervent Radiol 1987; 2: 9–13.

33. Busch E, Wilson PR. Atlanto-occipital and atlanto-axial injections in the treatment of headache and neck pain. Reg Anesth 1989; 14(Suppl. 2): 45.

34. Aprill C, Axinn MJ, Bogduk N. Occipital headaches stemming from the lateral atlanto-axial (C1–2) joint. Cephalalgia 2002; 22: 15–22.

35. Lord SM, Bogduk N. The cervical synovial joints as sources of post-traumatic headache. J Musculoskelet Pain 1996; 4: 81–94.

36. Kerr FWL: Trigeminal nerve volleys. Arch Neurol 1961; 5: 171–178.

37. Angus-Leppan H, Lambert GA, Michalicek J. Convergence of occipital nerve and superior sagittal sinus input in the cervical spinal cord of the cat. Cephalalgia 1997; 17: 625–630.

38. Bartsch T, Goadsby PJ. Stimulation of the greater occipital nerve induces increased central excitability of dural afferent input. Brain 2002; 125: 1496–1509.

39. Bartsch T, Goadsby PJ. Increased responses in trigeminocervical nociceptive neurons to cervical input after stimulation of the dura mater. Brain 2003; 126: 1801–1813.

40. Hu JW, Vernon H, Tatourian I. Changes in neck electromyography associated meningeal noxious stimulation. J Manipulative Physiol Ther 1995; 18: 577–581.

41. Giffin NJ, Ruggiero L, Lipton RB et al. Premonitory symptoms in migraine: an electronic diary study. Neurology 2003; 60: 935–940.

42. Goadsby PJ, Lipton RB, Ferrari MD. Migraine: current understanding and treatment. N Engl J Med 2002; 346: 257–270.

43. Bakal DA, Kaganov JA. Muscle contraction and migraine headache: psychologic comparison. Headache 1977; 17: 208–215.

44. Drummond PD. Scalp tenderness and sensitivity to pain in migraine and tension headache. Headache 1987; 27: 45–50.

45. Selby G, Lance JW. Observation on 500 cases of migraine and allied vascular headache. J Neurol Neurosurg Psychiatry 1960; 23: 23–32.

Cervicogenic headache: causes

In principle, pain can be caused in any of three ways. Nociceptive pain is caused by irritation of nerve endings in damaged or diseased structures. Neuropathic pain is caused by an intrinsic disorder of a peripheral nerve. Central pain is caused by a disturbance of pain pathways within the central nervous system.

The possible nociceptive causes of cervicogenic headache can be determined by taking the list of possible sources (Table 22.1) and, in effect, multiplying each by the possible lesions that can affect it. Some of these possible causes have been encountered in practice. Others remain conjectural or hypothetical.

Neuropathic causes of cervicogenic headache require a consideration of the disorders that might affect each or any of the upper three cervical nerves. Central pain is a conjectural entity in the context of cervicogenic headache.

NOCICEPTIVE PAIN

Arteries

Aneurysms of the vertebral artery and the internal carotid artery can cause pain, either in the head or the neck. Headache is the most common presenting feature of internal carotid artery dissection,[1,2] and may occur together with neck pain.[3] Headache is also the cardinal presenting feature of vertebral artery dissection. In both instances, some 60–70% of patients present with headache, typically in the occipital region, although not exclusively so.[1,3,4]

Aneurysms, therefore, are an important differential diagnosis of cervical causes of headache when the headache is acute, in either sense of the word (i.e. of recent onset or very severe). However, the rapid evolution of cerebrovascular symptoms and signs declares the nature of the condition. Consequently, aneurysm is not a differential diagnosis of chronic headache in the absence of cerebrovascular features.

A different concept related to arteries was proposed by Barré.[5] He maintained that headaches could be caused due to irritation of the vertebral nerve by arthritis of the cervical spine. The vertebral nerve is the sympathetic plexus that accompanies the vertebral artery. Others adopted or endorsed this contention and added that a whole host of cervical lesions could cause headache in this way.[6-11] By most of these authors, however, the mechanism of headache has never been more explicitly defined than "irritation of the vertebral nerve."

Table 22.1 The possible sources of cervicogenic headache, listed according to innervation and type of structure

Structure	Innervation		
	C1	C2	C3
Arteries	Vertebral; internal carotid		
Dura	Upper spinal cord; posterior cranial fossa		
Ligaments	Transverse atlanto-axial and alar; membrana tectoria		
Muscles	Prevertebral; sternocleidomastoid, trapezius		
	Suboccipital	Semispinalis, splenius	
			Multifidus; semispinalis
Joints	Median atlanto-axial		
	Atlanto-occipital	Lateral atlanto-axial	C2–3 zygapophysial
			C2–3 disc

Only Pawl[11] ventured to state that irritation of the vertebral nerve by cervical disc lesions or other lesions produces an autonomic barrage which results in spasm of the vertebrobasilar system, which produces head pain by causing ischemia of the vessel walls.

In both man and monkey, the so-called vertebral nerve consists of no more than gray rami communicantes accompanying the vertebral artery, and moreover, stimulation of these nerves or of the cervical sympathetic trunk in the monkey failed to influence vertebral blood flow.[12] Thus, neither anatomical nor physiological evidence was found which could support the vertebral nerve irritation theory. These experimental findings supported clinical opinion that there was no basis for belief in the Barré syndrome, otherwise known as migraine cervicale.[13,14]

Dura

The posterior cranial fossa is not commonly regarded as part of the neck. Consequently, diseases of the posterior fossa might not be considered intuitively as part of the differential diagnosis of headaches of cervical origin. However, since dura mater of the posterior cranial fossa is innervated by cervical nerves it falls within the neurological catchment area for cervical causes of headache. Diseases of the posterior cranial fossa, therefore, should not be neglected in the differential diagnosis. They include meningitis, meningeal irritation by blood after subarachnoid hemorrhage, and tumors that stretch the dura mater.

Ligaments

No studies have demonstrated that the ligaments of the upper cervical spine can be sources of cervicogenic headache. They remain only a theoretical source. Theoretically, sprain of the transverse or alar ligaments might cause pain. The involvement of these ligaments in rheumatoid arthritis is considered below, in the context of joint pain.

Muscles

There are no known diseases that affect muscles in a focal, localized manner to cause pain. Muscle diseases tend to be disseminated widely across individual muscles and across the body. Consequently, no muscle disease can be invoked as a cause of cervicogenic headache.

Some practitioners believe that sprains of muscles, or increased muscle tension, can be a cause of muscle pain. In the context of cervicogenic headache, however, no studies have established muscles to be the source of pain.

Many authors have asserted or endorsed that trigger points in the neck muscles can cause headache. The muscles implicated are the trapezius, sternocleidomastoid, and splenius capitis.[15-20] The diagnosis rests on finding by palpation the characteristic features of a trigger point. These are: a tender band within the muscle, which when palpated elicits a twitch response in the muscle, reproduces the patient's pain, and causes them to react— the so-called jump sign.[21]

In the context of neck pain and headache, this explanation of the cause of pain is difficult to sustain. Examination of the literature reveals that trigger points in the neck are exempt from the conventional diagnostic criteria. In the posterior neck muscles, instead of a palpable band, the trigger point is no more than a tender mass, from which a twitch response cannot be elicited.[22] No studies have demonstrated that the diagnosis of trigger points as a cause of headache is either reliable or valid. Conspicuously, these tender points typically overlie zygapophysial joints.[23] Therefore, they cannot be distinguished from underlying painful and tender joints.[23]

JOINTS

Neck tongue syndrome is a disorder characterized by acute unilateral occipital pain precipitated by sudden movement of the head, usually rotation, and accompanied by a sensation of numbness in the ipsilateral half of the tongue.[24] The pain appears to be caused by temporary subluxation of a lateral atlanto-axial joint, whereas the numbness of the tongue arises because of impingement, or stretching, of the C2 ventral ramus against the edge of the subluxated articular process.[25] The numbness occurs because proprioceptive afferents from the tongue pass from the ansa hypoglossi into the C2 ventral ramus.[24] Neck tongue syndrome can occur in patients with rheumatoid arthritis or with congenital joint laxity.[26] Hypomobility in the contralateral lateral atlanto-axial joint may predispose to the condition.[26]

Headache is a common feature of patients with *rheumatoid arthritis* of the upper cervical spine.[27–31] By inference, these headaches represent referred pain from inflamed atlanto-axial joints, and possibly from inflamed ligaments. Technically they constitute headache of cervical origin, but the distinctive circumstances in which they occur, in patients with overt rheumatoid arthritis, excludes them from the differential diagnosis of headache. Rheumatoid arthritis does not present with isolated headache. Rather, headache becomes a feature of patients with established rheumatoid arthritis when the disease extends to involve the C2 region.

Some authors have attributed headache to osteoarthritis of the median atlanto-axial joint.[32,33,34] The evidence for this association, however, is barely circumstantial. Whereas some patients with radiographically evident osteoarthritis do have occipital headache, others do not. The only statistical data pertain to an association between arthritic changes in the median atlanto-axial joint and suboccipital pain.[35] No such association has been demonstrated for headache. Detecting arthritis of the median atlanto-axial joint, therefore, is not diagnostic of a cervical source of

headache, for radiography alone cannot distinguish symptomatic osteoarthritic changes from asymptomatic age changes. A technique for verifying that a median atlanto-axial joint is painful has not been developed.

Headache has been noted in cases of congenital atlanto-axial dislocation, separation of the odontoid, and occipitalization of the atlas.[36,37] There is no evidence, however, that these abnormalities, *per se*, are symptomatic. Indeed, they can be asymptomatic. Their presence and identification does not provide a diagnosis. They may predispose to mechanical disorders of the neck, but they may be totally incidental findings.

Stimulation of the *atlanto-occipital joints* has been shown to cause headache in normal volunteers, but this observation has still not been complemented by studies that show that these joints are the source of pain in patients with headache. Consequently, it is not known how commonly the atlanto-occipital joints are a source of cervicogenic headache.

Studies in normal volunteers have shown that noxious stimulation of the lateral atlanto-axial joint can produce referred pain to the head.[38] Clinical studies have shown that headache can be relieved by anesthetizing this joint.[39–42] There would appear, therefore, to be sufficient evidence to implicate the lateral atlanto-axial joint as one possible cervical source of headache. No studies, however, have established what the pathology might be. One study attributed the pain to radiographically evident osteoarthritis,[39] but such arthritis is not always evident. A post-mortem study has indicated that, in post-traumatic cases, the responsible lesions might include capsular rupture, intra-articular hemorrhage, and bruising of intra-articular meniscoids, or small fractures through the superior articular process of the axis.[43]

The prevalence of lateral atlanto-axial joint pain is not known, but it may not be uncommon. One study traced the source of pain to the lateral atlanto-axial joints in 16% of patients presenting with headache, but not all patients were investigated for this condition, which suggests that 16% may be an underestimate.[42]

Diagnostic blocks are the only means of establishing the diagnosis. They involve injecting a small volume of local anesthetic into the joint, under fluoroscopic guidance. Certain clinical features may be suggestive of lateral atlanto-axial joint pain, but they are not diagnostic in their own right. These include: pain in the occipital or suboccipital region, together with maximal or focal tenderness in the suboccipital region, maximal or focal tenderness over the tip of the left or right transverse process of C1, restricted rotation of C1 on C2 on manual examination of that segment, and aggravation of the patient's accustomed headache by passive rotation of the C1 vertebra to the left or right.[42]

The *C2–3 zygapophysial joint* is innervated by the third occipital nerve. Headache stemming from the C2–3 zygapophysial joint, therefore, can be relieved by third occipital nerve blocks, and accordingly has been named third occipital headache.

Initial studies describing third occipital headache were conducted using single diagnostic blocks with no controls.[44,45] A subsequent study used controlled diagnostic blocks and confirmed the existence of this entity.[46] Moreover, that study established the prevalence of third occipital headache. In patients with headache after whiplash, the prevalence of third occipital headache was 27%. Among patients in whom headache was the dominant complaint, the prevalence was 53% (95% CI: 37%, 68%).

There are no clinical features that are diagnostic of third occipital headache. Tenderness over the C2–3 joint is suggestive, but has a positive likelihood ratio of only 2.1.[46] Controlled diagnostic blocks are the only means of establishing the diagnosis with confidence.[46]

There is some evidence to implicate the C2–3 *intervertebral disc* as a source of cervicogenic headache. Stimulation of this disc reproduces the pain suffered by some patients with headache.[47,48] Arthrodesis of that disc has been reported to relieve headache.[49] The nature of the causative pathology remains unknown.

Zygapophysial joints below C2–3 can sometimes be a source of headache, but their prevalence decreases rapidly the further they are displaced from the C2–3 segment and the C1, 2, 3 nerves.[50]

NEUROPATHIC PAIN

Occipital neuralgia is an ill-defined entity that has been invoked as a cause of cervicogenic headache. The term implies some sort of disorder of the greater occipital nerve.

The International Association for the Study of Pain (IASP) defines *occipital neuralgia* as "pain, usually deep and aching, in the distribution of the second cervical dorsal root."[51] The International Headache Society (IHS) defines it as "paroxysmal jabbing pain in the distribution of the greater or lesser occipital nerves, accompanied by diminished sensation or dysesthesia in the affected area."[52] However, although the IHS stipulates sensory abnormalities in its definition, these are not listed among the diagnostic criteria.

These definitions differ in one critical respect; the IHS stipulates that the pain must be paroxysmal and jabbing, whereas the IASP describes it as deep and aching pain, and only sometimes stabbing in nature. The IASP states that "nerve block may give relief," but the IHS insists that temporary relief by anesthetic block is a mandatory diagnostic criterion.

This inconsistency, conflict and contradiction are characteristic of the literature on occipital neuralgia. There is no consensus on definition or diagnostic criteria, and the rubric is used loosely if not arbitrarily to refer to any pain felt in the occipital region.

The term "neuralgia" explicitly means pain stemming from a nerve, and should be reserved for such conditions. Paroxysmal lancinating pain is the hallmark of neuralgia and should be an essential diagnostic criterion for occipital neuralgia, if that term is to be used. In this respect the definition of the IASP is in error. Deep, aching pain in the occiput can arise from a variety of sources and causes, not the least of which are diseases of the posterior cranial fossa and base of skull[53] and the upper cervical joints.[39–42,44–46] Indeed, the IHS comments that occipital neuralgia must be distinguished from occipital referral of pain from the atlanto-axial or upper zygapophysial joints.[52]

The IASP definition would include these latter conditions even though they do not involve irritation or compression of the greater occipital nerve or even the C2 spinal nerve. Deep, aching pain in the occiput is not indicative of irritation of the greater occipital nerve. It is no more than a protean symptom, for which a specific cause should be found. The habit of attributing such pain to irritation of the greater occipital nerve stems from an era when neurologists and neurosurgeons were oblivious to somatic referred pain, and ascribed any and every pain to irritation of a nerve.

There is no compelling evidence that occipital pain is due to irritation of the greater occipital nerve. Lancinating occipital neuralgia has been recorded as a feature of *temporal arteritis*,[54] in which case inflammation of occipital artery could affect the companion nerve. However, in the majority of cases of so-called occipital neuralgia no such pathology is evident.

The commonly held view is that occipital neuralgia is caused by entrapment of the greater occipital nerve where it pierces trapezius. Surgical studies do not provide circumstantial evidence of this. Liberation of the nerve initially relieves headache in some 80% of cases but the relief has a median duration of only some 3–6 months.[55] Excision of the greater occipital nerve provides relief in some 70% of patients, but this has a median duration of only 244 days.[56]

The cardinal diagnostic criterion seems to be response to blocks of the greater occipital nerve; but these blocks are not target-specific when they involve volumes such as 5 ml[55] or 10 ml.[57,58] In such volumes they do not selectively implicate the greater occipital nerve. No studies using more discrete blocks have implicated the greater occipital nerve as the source of pain.

A distinctive form of headache known as *C2 neuralgia* can be caused by lesions affecting the C2 spinal nerve.

This nerve runs behind the lateral atlanto-axial joint, resting on its capsule.[25,59] Inflammatory or other disorders of the joint may result in the nerve becoming incorporated in the fibrotic changes of chronic inflammation.[60,61] Release of the nerve relieves the symptoms. Otherwise, the C2 spinal nerve and its roots are surrounded by a sleeve of dura mater and a plexus of epiradicular veins, lesions of which can compromise the nerve. These include meningioma,[62] neurinoma[61] and anomalous vertebral arteries;[63] but the majority of reported cases have involved venous abnormalities ranging from single to densely interwoven, dilated veins surrounding the C2 spinal nerve and its roots[64] to U-shaped arterial loops or angiomas compressing the C2 dorsal root ganglion.[60,64,65]

Nerves affected by vascular abnormalities exhibit a variety of features indicative of neuropathy, such as myelin breakdown, chronic hemorrhage, axon degeneration and regeneration and increased endoneurial and pericapsular connective tissue.[64] It is not clear, however, whether the vascular abnormality causes these neuropathic changes or is only coincident with them.

C2 neuralgia is characterized by intermittent, lancinating pain in the occipital region associated with lacrimation and ciliary injection. The pain typically occurs in association with a background of dull occipital pain and dull, referred pain in the temporal, frontal and orbital regions. Most often, this latter pain is focused on the fronto-orbital region, but encompasses all three regions when severe. However, the distinguishing feature of this condition is a cutting or tearing sensation in the occipital region, which is the hallmark of its neurogenic basis. In this regard, C2 neuralgia probably represents what previously had been called occipital neuralgia as defined by the International Headache Society.[52]

C2 neuralgia is distinguished from referred pain from the neck by its neurogenic quality, its periodicity, and its association with lacrimation and ciliary injection. The latter association has attracted the appellation of "cluster-like" headache.[62] The cardinal diagnostic feature is complete relief of pain following local anesthetic blockade of the suspected nerve root—typically the C2 spinal nerve, but occasionally the C3 nerve. These blocks are performed under radiological control and employ discrete amounts (0.6–0.8 ml) of long-acting local anesthetic to block the target nerve selectively.[60]

CENTRAL PAIN

The causes of primary headaches, such as migraine and tension-type headache, still remain unknown. One concept that has been invoked to explain their mechanism is dysnociception.[66] The concept postulates that disturbances occur in nuclei that regulate the trigeminocervical nucleus, resulting in disinhibition of the nucleus. As a result, the patient perceives pain because of increased activity in central trigeminocervical neurons. That activity, however, is effectively spontaneous. The cells are not activated by nociceptive activity arriving along trigeminal or cervical afferents. The source of the pain is wholly within the central nervous system.

It is possible that cervicogenic headache could be caused by such a mechanism. Indeed, it has been recognized as a possibility,[67] but it is no more than a theoretical concept. No actual evidence implicates such a mechanism. Nevertheless, it is a threat to other interpretations of cervicogenic headache. Various signs used to diagnose cervicogenic headache, even diagnostic

Table 22.2 The possible causes of cervicogenic headache, tabulated by mechanism and whether or not the cause and source can be demonstrated

Mechanism	Demonstrable source Known cause	Demonstrable source Cause unknown	Conjectural, No evidence
Nociceptive			
	Aneurysms: —vertebral artery —internal carotid artery Meningitis Tumors of posterior cranial fossa	Lateral atlanto-axial joint C2–3 zygapophysial joint C2–3 disc	Median atlanto-axial joint Atlanto-occipital joint Ligament sprain Muscle tension
Neuropathic			
	C2 neuralgia		Occipital neuralgia
Central			
			Dysnociception

blocks, might all be reflections of central hyperalgesia rather than valid features of a peripheral (and cervical) source of pain.

SYNOPSIS

The possible causes of cervicogenic headache can be tabulated according to mechanism and whether the source can be demonstrated, whether the cause is known, or whether the cause is only conjectural and not supported by evidence (Table 22.2). A central mechanism remains totally conjectural. Of the neuropathic mechanisms, C2 neuralgia has a demonstrable source and known causes, but there is sufficient evidence to render occipital neuralgia as a valid cause. Most of the causes are nociceptive.

Aneurysms and diseases of the posterior cranial fossa are identifiable causes, but are fortunately rare. For common presentations of cervicogenic headache, the strongest available evidence implicates the lateral atlanto-axial joints, the C2–3 zygapophysial joint, and the C2–3 disc as the likely sources of pain; but evidence is lacking as to the actual cause of pain. Clinical evidence is lacking that cervicogenic headache stems from the ligaments or muscles of the upper cervical spine, or from the atlanto-occipital or median atlanto-axial joints.

References

1. Silbert PL, Makri B, Schievink WI. Headache and neck pain in spontaneous internal carotid and vertebral artery dissections. Neurology 1995; 45: 1517–1522.
2. Biousse V, D'Anglejan-Chatillon J, Massiou H, Bousser MG. Head pain in non-traumatic carotid artery dissection: a series of 65 patients. Cephalalgia 1994; 14: 33–36.
3. Sturzenegger M. Headache and neck pain: the warning symptoms of vertebral artery dissection. Headache 1994; 34: 187–193.
4. Mokri B, Houser W, Sandok BA, Piepgras DG. Spontaneous dissections of the vertebral arteries. Neurology 1988; 38: 880–885.
5. Barre N. Sur un syndrome sympathique cervicale posterieure et sa cause frequente: l'arthrite cervicale. Revue du Neurologie 1926; 33: 1246–1248.
6. Gayral L, Neuwirth E. Oto-neuro-opthalmologic manifestations of cervical origin: posterior cervical sympathetic syndrome of Barre-Lieou. NY State J Med 1954; 54: 1920–1926.
7. Neuwirth E. Neurologic complications of osteoarthritis of the cervical spine. NY State J Med 1954; 54: 2583–2590.
8. Kovacs A. Subluxation and deformation of the cervical apophyseal joints. Acta Radiol 1955; 43: 1–16.
9. Stewart DY. Current concepts of "Barre syndrome" or the "posterior cervical sympathetic syndrome." Clin Orthop 1962; 24: 40–48.
10. Dutton CD, Riley LH. Cervical migraine: not merely a pain in the neck. Am J Med 1969;47: 141–148.
11. Pawl RP. Headache, cervical spondylosis, and anterior cervical fusion. Surg Ann 1977; 9: 391–408.
12. Bogduk N, Lambert G, Duckworth JW. The anatomy and physiology of the vertebral nerve in relation to cervical migraine. Cephalalgia 1981; 1: 1–14.
13. Bartschi-Rochaix W. Headaches of cervical origin. In: Vinken PJ, Bruyn GW (eds). Handbook of Clinical Neurology. Elsevier, New York, 1968, 5: 192–203.
14. Lance JW. Mechanism and Management of Headache, 4th edn. Butterworths, London, 1982.
15. Travell J, Rinzler SH. The myofascial genesis of pain. Postgrad Med 1952; 11: 425–434.
16. Travell J. Mechanical headache. Headache 1962; 7: 23–29.
17. Travell J. Referred pain from skeletal muscle: the pectoralis major syndrome of breast pain and soreness and the sternomastoid syndrome of headache and dizziness. NY State J Med 1955; 55: 331–340.
18. Bonica JJ. Management of myofascial pain syndromes in general practice. JAMA 1957; 164: 732–738.
19. Berges PU. Myofascial pain syndromes. Postgrad Med 1973; 53: 161–168.
20. Rubin D. Myofascial trigger point syndromes: an approach to management. Arch Phys Med Rehabil 1981; 62: 107–110.
21. Simons DG. Myofascial pain syndromes; where are we; where are we going? Arch Phys Med Rehabil 1988; 69: 207–212.
22. Travell JG, Simons DG. Myofascial Pain and Dysfunction: The Trigger Point Manual. Williams and Wilkins, Baltimore, 1993: 312.
23. Bogduk N, Simons DG. Neck pain: joint pain or trigger points. In: Vaeroy H, Merskey H (eds). Progress in Fibromyalgia and Myofascial Pain. Elsevier, Amsterdam, 1993: 267–273.
24. Lance JW, Anthony M. Neck tongue syndrome on sudden turning of the head. J Neurol Neurosurg Psychiat 1980; 43: 97–101.
25. Bogduk N. An anatomical basis for neck tongue syndrome. J Neurol Neurosurg Psychiat 1981; 44: 202–208.
26. Bertoft ES, Westerberg CE. Further observations on the neck-tongue syndrome. Cephalalgia 1985; 5(Suppl. 3):312–313.
27. Bland JH, Davis PH, London MG et al. Rheumatoid arthritis of the cervical spine. Arch Int Med 1963; 112: 892–898.
28. Cabot A, Becker A. The cervical spine in rheumatoid arthritis. Clin Orthop 1978; 131: 130–140.
29. Robinson, HS. Rheumatoid arthritis: atlanto-axial subluxation and its clinical presentation. Can Med Ass J 1966; 94: 470–477.
30. Sharp J, Purser DW. Spontaneous atlanto-axial dislocation in ankylosing spondylitis and rheumatoid arthritis. Ann Rheum Dis 1961; 20: 47–77.
31. Stevens JS, Cartlidge NEF, Saunders M, Appleby A, Hall M, Shaw DA. Atlanto-axial subluxation and cervical myelopathy in rheumatoid arthritis. Quart J Med 1971; 159: 391–408.
32. Fournier AM, Rathelot P. L'Arthrose atlo-odontoidienne. La Presse Medicale 1960; 68:163–165.
33. Harata S, Tohno S, Kawagishi T. Osteoarthritis of the atlanto-axial joint. Int Orthop 1981; 5: 277–282.
34. Zapletal J, Hekster REM, Straver JS, Wilmink JT. Atlanto-odontoid osteoarthritis: appearance prevalence at computed tomography. Spine 1995; 20: 49–53.
35. Zapletal J, Hekster REM, Straver JS, Wilmink JT, Hermans J. Relationship between atlanto-odontoid osteoarthritis and idiopathic suboccipital neck pain. Neuroradiology 1996; 38: 62–65.
36. McRae DL. The significance of abnormalities of the cervical spine. AJR 1960; 84: 3–25.
37. McRae DL. Bony abnormalities of the cranio-spinal junction. Clin Neurosurg 1968; 16: 356–375.
38. Dreyfuss P, Michaelsen M, Fletcher D. Atlanto-occipital and lateral atlanto-axial joint pain patterns. Spine 1994; 19: 1125–1131.

39. Ehni G, Benner B. Occipital neuralgia and the C1–2 arthrosis syndrome. J Neurosurg 1984; 61: 961–965.

40. McCormick CC. Arthrography of the atlanto-axial (C1–C2) joints: technique and results. J Intervent Radiol 1987; 2: 9–13.

41. Busch E, Wilson PR. Atlanto-occipital and atlanto-axial injections in the treatment of headache and neck pain. Reg Anesth 1989, 14(Suppl. 2): 45.

42. Aprill C, Axinn MJ, Bogduk N. Occipital headaches stemming from the lateral atlanto-axial (C1–2) joint. Cephalalgia 2002; 22: 15–22.

43. Schonstrom N, Twomey L, Taylor J. The lateral atlanto-axial joints and their synovial folds: an in vitro study of soft tissue injuries and fractures. J Trauma 1993; 35: 886–892.

44. Bogduk N, Marsland A. On the concept of third occipital headache. J Neurol Neurosurg Psychiat 1986; 49: 775–780.

45. Bogduk N, Marsland A. The cervical zygapophysial joints as a source of neck pain. Spine 1988; 13: 610–617.

46. Lord S, Barnsley L, Wallis B, Bogduk N. Third occipital headache: a prevalence study. J Neurol Neurosurg Psychiat 1994; 57: 1187–1190.

47. Schellhas KP, Smith MD, Gundry CR, Pollei SR. Cervical discogenic pain: prospective correlation of magnetic resonance imaging and discography in asymptomatic subjects and pain sufferers. Spine 1996; 21: 300–312.

48. Grubb SA, Kelly CK. Cervical discography: clinical implications from 12 years of experience. Spine 2000; 25: 1382–1389.

49. Schofferman J, Garges K, Goldthwaite N, Kosetler M, Libby E. Upper cervical anterior diskectomy and fusion improves discogenic cervical headaches. Spine 2002; 27: 2240–2244.

50. Lord SM, Bogduk N. The cervical synovial joints as sources of post-traumatic headache. J Musculoskel Pain 1996; 4: 81–94.

51. Merskey H, Bogduk N (eds). Classification of Pain: Descriptions of Chronic Pain Syndromes and Definitions of Pain Terms, 2nd edn. International Association for the Study of Pain, Seattle, 1994: 64–65.

52. Headache Classification Committee of the International Headache Society. Classification and Diagnostic Criteria for Headache Disorders, Cranial Neuralgias and Facial Pain. Cephalalgia 1988; 8(Suppl. 7): 1–96.

53. Sigwald J, Jamet F. Occipital neuralgia. In: Vinken PJ, Bruyn GW (eds). Handbook of Clinical Neurology. Elsevier, New York, 1968, 5: 368–374.

54. Jundt JW, Mock D. Temporal arteritis with normal erythrocyte sediment rates presenting as occipital neuralgia. Arthritis Rheum 1991; 34: 217–219.

55. Bovim G, Fredriksen TA, Stolt-Nielsen A, Sjaastad O. Neurolysis of the greater occipital nerve in cervicogenic headache: a follow up study. Headache 1992; 32: 175–179.

56. Anthony M. Headache and the greater occipital nerve. Clin Neurol Neurosurg 1992; 94: 297–301.

57. Saadah HA, Taylor FB. Sustained headache syndrome associated with tender occipital nerve zones. Headache 1987; 27: 201–205.

58. Gawel MJ, Rothbart PJ. Occipital nerve block in the management of headache and cervical pain. Cephalalgia 1992; 12: 9–13.

59. Bogduk N. Local anaesthetic blocks of the second cervical ganglion: a technique with application in occipital headache. Cephalalgia 1981; 1: 41–50.

60. Jansen J, Markakis E, Rama B, Hildebrandt J. Hemicranial attacks or permanent hemicrania: a sequel of upper cervical root compression. Cephalalgia 1989; 9: 123–130.

61. Poletti CE, Sweet WH. Entrapment of the C2 root and ganglion by the atlanto-epistrophic ligament: clinical syndrome and surgical anatomy. Neurosurgery 1990; 27: 288–291.

62. Kuritzky, A. Cluster headache-like pain caused by an upper cervical meningioma. Cephalalgia 1984; 4: 185–186.

63. Sharma RR, Parekh HC, Prabhu S, Gurusinghe NT, Bertolis G. Compression of the C2 root by a rare anomalous ectatic vertebral artery. J Neurosurg 1993; 78: 669–672.

64. Jansen J, Bardosi A, Hildebrandt J, Lucke A. Cervicogenic, hemicranial attacks associated with vascular irritation or compression of the cervical nerve root C2. Clinical manifestations and morphological findings. Pain 1989; 39: 203–212.

65. Hildebrandt J, Jansen J. Vascular compression of the C2 and C3 roots: yet another cause of chronic intermittent hemicrania? Cephalalgia 1984; 4: 167–170.

66. Olesen J, Langemark M. Mechanism of tension headache: a speculative hypothesis. In: Olesen J, Edvinsson L (eds). Basic Mechanisms of Headache. Pain Research and Clinical Management. Elsevier, Amsterdam, 1988, 2: 457–461.

67. Bogduk N. Headache and the neck. In: Goadsby PJ, Silberstein SD (eds). Headache. Butterworth-Heinemann, Boston, 1997: 369–381.

23 Cervicogenic headache: diagnosis

> ## KEY POINTS
>
> - Proposed clinical criteria for the diagnosis of cervicogenic headache lack validity.
>
> - Manual examination also lacks validity and is possibly unreliable.
>
> - Nonetheless, clinical assessment can be used to suspect cervicogenic headache, and to formulate a diagnosis of *possible* and *probable* cervicogenic headache.
>
> - The definitive diagnosis of cervicogenic headache requires controlled diagnostic blocks of the structure believed to be the source of pain, or its nerve supply.

Three approaches have been used to diagnose cervicogenic headache. Headache specialists have pursued a clinical approach. Manual therapists have used manual examination. Pain specialists have advocated diagnostic blocks.

CLINICAL

It has been traditional to define primary headaches on the basis of their clinical features. This approach to nosology arose because the various primary headaches were recognized as clinical entities well before anything was understood about their pathology, and no objective biological marker, such as a blood test or imaging test, distinguished them. The convention became to define these entities in terms of: location of pain, frequency, periodicity, precipitating factors, aggravating factors, relieving factors, and associated features. That convention remains in force for accepted entities such as migraine, cluster headache, and tension-type headache, and has been applied to more recently recognized entities such as paroxysmal hemicrania and SUNCT (Short-lasting, Unilateral, Neuralgiform headache attacks with Conjunctival injection and Tearing).

It should not be surprising, therefore, that proponents of a new entity would follow this convention. Accordingly, authorities intent on promoting cervicogenic headache as a new and distinct entity elected to define it according to clinical features.

Criteria

Preliminary diagnostic criteria for cervicogenic headache were developed in 1987,[1] and were consolidated into a formal statement in 1990.[2] The criteria encompassed certain "major criteria," certain characteristics of the pain, other "important" criteria, and a list of minor criteria that were considered not obligatory (Table 23.1). Obligatory for the diagnosis were: unilateral head pain without side-shift, and symptoms or signs of cervical involvement. For the latter, at least one of the listed features was obligatory, namely provocation of pain

Table 23.1 The diagnostic criteria for cervicogenic headache, as proposed in 1990[2] and as amended in 1998.[3] The major amendments are indicated by an asterisk*

	1990 Criteria		**1998 Criteria**
MAJOR			
I	Unilateral	III	Unilateral
II	Cervical involvement	*I	Cervical involvement
a	Provocation:	a	Precipitation of pain
1	by neck movement or sustained posture	1	by neck movement or sustained posture
2	by external pressure	2	by external pressure
b	Neck, shoulder, and arm pain	b	Neck, shoulder, or arm pain
c	Reduced range of motion	c	Restricted range of motion
		*II	Anesthetic blockade
PAIN			
III	Non-clustering	IV c	Fluctuating, continuous
IV	Varying duration	IV b	Varying duration
V	Moderate pain, usually not throbbing	IV a	Moderate-severe, not throbbing, not lancinating,
VI	Pain starts in neck		Starting in the neck
OTHER			
VII	Anesthetic blocks abolish pain		
VIII	Female	V c	Female
IX	History of head or neck trauma	V d	History of head or neck trauma
		V a	Lack effect of indometacin
		V b	Lack effect ergotamine, sumatriptan
MINOR			
X	Nausea, vomiting, edema	VI a	Nausea
XI	Dizziness	VI c	Dizziness
XII	Phonophobia, photophobia	VI b	Phonophobia, photophobia
XIII	Blurred vision	VI d	Blurred vision
XIV	Difficulties swallowing	VI e	Difficulties swallowing
		VI f	Edema

by neck movement or by external pressure to the upper posterior neck; or concurrent neck pain; or reduced range of motion of the neck. It was considered that one—or preferably two—of the characteristics of the pain should also apply, although this was not obligatory. Similarly, it was desirable but not obligatory that at least one of the other important criteria apply.

Applying these criteria, as recommended, yields a rather contentious entity. This is unilateral headache, provoked by neck movement or by palpation of the neck, OR associated with neck pain or reduced range of movement, PERHAPS of varying duration, PERHAPS moderate in intensity and not throbbing, PERHAPS starting in the neck, PERHAPS following trauma, and PERHAPS relieved by anesthetic blocks.

Restricting the definition to only the obligatory criteria amounts to unilateral headache with a hint of an abnormality in the cervical spine.

Challenges

Following the publication of these criteria, several studies examined their specificity. They were prompted by the perception that the proposed features were shared by other, established entities, and were not diagnostic of a unique type of headache.

One group of investigators[4,5,6] assessed the specificity of unilaterality without side-shift. In various samples they found that this feature occurred in 17%,[4] 20%,[5] and over 30%[6] of patients with migraine, and in up to 20% of patients with tension-type headache.[6] A subsequent review reiterated these findings and added that triggering of headache by neck movement or by pressure on the neck were uncommon findings among patients with headache.[7] The review found that the prevalence of neck pain associated with headache could be no more than a coincidence given how common each of these complaints is in the general community.

Other studies examined particular features. As a group, patients believed to have cervicogenic headache exhibited reduced pressure-pain thresholds, compared with normal controls, patients with migraine and patients with tension-type headache.[8] Patients with presumed cervicogenic headache exhibited a variety of impairments of cervical muscle function.[9] In both instances, however, the distribution of scores in the patients overlapped considerably that of normal subjects, so that a valid diagnostic criterion could not be supported.

One study found no significant radiographic abnormalities of the head or cervical spine in patients with cervicogenic headache.[10] Another found no differences between patients with cervicogenic headache and normal subjects, with respect to morphologic abnormalities on radiographs of the neck or radiographic

hypomobility of the neck.[11] A more detailed radiographic study found no differences from normal in the range of lateral flexion of the neck in patients with cervicogenic headache, but did find significant reduction in the range of axial rotation and flexion-extension.[12] However, the ranges of values exhibited by the headache patients overlapped those of patients with migraine or tension-type headache, and those of normal controls. Consequently, a clinically useful and valid threshold of abnormality could not be derived.

These observations seriously challenged the specificity of the original criteria for cervicogenic headache. Individual features such as unilaterality, provocation by neck movement or digital pressure on the neck, impaired muscle function, and reduced range of movement did not constitute discriminating criteria.

Responses

The challenges to validity of cervicogenic headache as a nosological entity were met in two ways. First, the diagnostic criteria were revised. Second, several studies were conducted to test the reliability and validity of the criteria.

Several amendments to the criteria were announced in 1998[3] (Table 23.1). Foremost, evidence of cervical involvement was promoted to the first of the major criteria. Unilaterality was demoted to the third of the major criteria. Furthermore, the unilaterality criterion was relaxed. It was stated that, in the typical case, pain is unilateral, but may spread across the midline during episodes of severe pain, still with a preponderance on the usual side. As well, bilateral headache was accepted for routine work (as opposed to scientific work), but with the warning to distinguish such patients from those with tension headache.

Promoted to a major criterion was response to anesthetic blockade of the greater or lesser occipital nerve, the C2 spinal nerve, the third occipital nerve, the cervical zygapophysial joints, or lower cervical nerve roots. The required effect was defined as: "the pain is drastically reduced."

Otherwise, the criteria concerning the characteristics of the pain were renumbered but remained unchanged. The minor, non-obligatory criteria were expanded to include lack of response to ergotamine, sumatriptan, and indometacin.

These revised criteria were tested for reliability. The results of the study were reported in two papers.[13,14] The earlier report is the more comprehensive, and described the agreement achieved by various neurologists and anesthesiologists.[13] The second paper reprised the same study, but reported only on the results of physical examination, and only the results achieved by the two expert neurologists engaged in the first study.[14]

For agreement on a diagnosis of cervicogenic headache, the kappa scores ranged from 0.43 to 0.83.[13] Qualitatively, these scores represent fair to very good agreement. Higher scores were obtained between expert neurologists and expert anesthesiologists accustomed to diagnosing cervicogenic headache. Among the clinical features, the most reliable were "pain starts in the neck and radiates to the fronto-temporal region," "pain radiates to the ipsilateral shoulder and arm," "nausea," "vomiting," "photophobia," and "phonophobia." Among the physical examination features, the most reliable was "provocation of pain by neck movement." Other features, such as "restricted range of motion" and "pressure pain on palpation" had unacceptably low agreement. In the second paper,[14] better agreement was reported. The feature "provocation of pain by neck movement" remained the most reliable sign; and "pressure pain on palpation" achieved acceptable agreement. The other features retained fair or poor agreement.

A study published in only a short form[15] assessed the validity of the original criteria for distinguishing cervicogenic headache from migraine and tension-type headache. The author reported the percentages of patients with each type of headache that fulfilled various criteria, but did not provide any tabulated data. Therefore, readers cannot undertake an incisive analysis. Nevertheless, one feature that emerged was that patients with cervicogenic headache could be distinguished from those with migraine or tension type headache if they satisfied at least seven of the diagnostic criteria. This observation heralded the importance of requiring multiple simultaneous criteria for the diagnosis.

Another group pursued this theme.[16] They reduced the revised criteria[3] to a list of seven criteria (Box 23.1). They also qualified the certainty of diagnosis. They proposed that two criteria provided an initial step to identify patients with *possible* cervicogenic headache. Those were: unilateral headache, and pain starting in the neck. Satisfying any three additional criteria promoted the diagnosis to *probable* cervicogenic headache.

Using these operational guidelines, the authors felt that they could confidently distinguish cervicogenic headache from migraine. Only 17% of their patients satisfied both the diagnostic criteria for cervicogenic headache as proposed by the authors and the criteria for migraine proposed by the International Headache Society.[17] The clinical features most strongly indicative of cervicogenic headache were: "pain radiating to the shoulder and arm," "varying duration or fluctuating continuous pain," "moderate, non-throbbing pain," and "history of neck trauma."

BOX 23.1
THE COLLAPSED CRITERIA FOR CERVICOGENIC HEADACHE[16]

1. Unilateral headache without side-shift
2. Symptoms and signs of neck involvement:
   pain triggered by neck movement or sustained awkward posture and/or external pressure of the posterior neck or occipital region
   ipsilateral neck, shoulder, and arm pain
   reduced range of motion
3. Pain episodes of varying duration or fluctuating continuous pain
4. Moderate, non-excruciating pain, usually of a non-throbbing nature
5. Pain starting in the neck, spreading to oculo-fronto-temporal areas
6. Anesthetic blockades abolish the pain transiently provided complete anesthesia is obtained
   or
   sustained neck trauma a relatively short time prior to the onset
7. Various attack-related phenomena: autonomic symptoms and signs, nausea, vomiting, ispilateral edema and flushing in the periocular area, dizziness, photophobia, phonophobia, blurred vision in the ipsilateral eye.

Conflicts

Although investigators have sought to defend the diagnostic criteria for cervicogenic headache, they have examined only the nosologic validity of the criteria, i.e. the extent to which the criteria seem to distinguish cervicogenic headache from migraine and tension-type headache. No studies have established that patients who satisfy the diagnostic criteria actually have a cervical source for their pain.

Fundamental to the concept of cervicogenic headache is that it constitutes pain referred to the head from a cervical source. Therefore, demonstrating such a source is essential for the diagnosis.

Clinical features alone are not enough to demonstrate a cervical source of pain. Even among proponents of cervicogenic headache, the inter-observer reliability for most clinical signs is variable.[13] It is lacking, or at best fair, for restricted range of motion, tenderness over the zygapophysial joints, and tenderness over the occiput. In expert hands, it is moderate for provocation of pain by neck movement, and for pressure over the posterior border of the sternocleidomastoid muscle.[14] Yet even the proponents acknowledge that: "it is highly questionable whether such satisfactory results could be obtained by physicians who were not experienced at diagnosing headache syndromes." Even if reliability is accepted, there is no evidence that any of these features are valid signs of a cervical disorder. Nor has radiography revealed any signs of a cervical lesion.[10,11]

In essence and in effect, the "clinical" approach to defining cervicogenic headache has not succeeded to date.

MANUAL EXAMINATION

Manual therapists contend that they can identify symptomatic joints in the cervical spine by specialized manual examination. In particular, they base their assessment on examining passive accessory intersegmental movements, and the reproduction of pain during this testing.

The validity of this approach to diagnosis rests on one small study. It reported that a manual therapist was very accurate at identifying zygapophysial joints found to be painful by diagnostic, local anesthetic blocks of the joint.[18] Those results, however, cannot be generalized. In its discussion, the study called for replication studies to show either or both that other manual therapists were just as accurate and that manual therapists could agree on their palpatory findings.

No subsequent studies of validity have eventuated in the 20 years since that first study. Two studies of reliability found manual examination of passive accessory intersegmental movements of the cervical spine to be unreliable, with kappa scores of less than 0.40.[19,20] Another study claimed that manual therapists were, indeed, able to agree on whether an atlanto-occipital, atlanto-axial, or C2–3 zygapophysial joint was symptomatic in patients with headache.[21] That study was criticized for not providing enough data by which the calculation of kappa scores could be checked,[22] but the challenge to provide those data was declined.[23] Technically, therefore, the purported skills of manual therapists remain unproven, with the available evidence suggesting that the assessment techniques that they use are not reliable.

In the most recent study of manual therapy for headaches,[24] manual examination was performed, but the diagnosis of cervicogenic headache was established essentially on the basis of the proposed clinical criteria.[2,3] Accordingly, it seems that manual therapists are reluctant to base their diagnosis exclusively on manual assessment.

DIAGNOSTIC BLOCKS

A third approach to the diagnosis of cervicogenic headache was foreshadowed in an editorial in 1984.[24] That editorial listed the criteria that should be satisfied

---

BOX 23.2
SUGGESTED CRITERIA FOR ESTABLISHING A CERVICAL SOURCE FOR HEADACHE[24]

1. Stimulation of some structure in the neck should evoke the headache
2. Where possible, anesthetization of that structure should promptly relieve the headache
3. The location of the pain-producing focus should be specified in anatomical terms
4. The pathology of the focus should be defined.

---

for a cervical cause for headache to be credited (Box 23.2).

The editorial recognized that the fourth criterion might be hard to satisfy, for it depended on high-resolution imaging techniques that might not be available. They remain lacking to this day. However, the editorial argued that the judicious and disciplined application of diagnostic blocks would satisfy criteria 2 and 3.

Response to anesthetic blocks was mentioned in the original criteria for cervicogenic headache (Table 23.1), but this criterion was not prominent; the emphasis was on "clinical" features. Subsequently, although "anesthetic blockade" was promoted to a major criterion in the revised criteria (Table 23.1), it has not been widely adopted by proponents of cervicogenic headache. Indeed, in the collapsed criteria (Box 23.1), an alternative to "response to anesthetic blocks" as a criterion is "history of trauma." It would seem that local anesthetic blocks are given lip-service but remain overshadowed by a predilection with "clinical" features.

In the few studies in which blocks have been undertaken, the standard of practice has been less than ideal, and the results mixed. In one study, blocks of the greater occipital nerve were performed in 22 patients with suspected cervicogenic headache, using 1.5 ml of 2% lidocaine.[25] Fourteen patients had control blocks with normal saline, which provided no relief. Following the active blocks, seven of the 22 patients had complete relief of headache; a further three had nearly complete relief; seven had 50% relief; and the remainder had partial or no relief. Responses were assessed for only 30 minutes.

These results are difficult to interpret. Complete relief of pain is an attractive response, but it occurred in less than half of the cases. One interpretation is that these patients had pain mediated by the greater occipital nerve. The other patients either did not have cervicogenic headache or if they did, the source of pain was not in the territory of the greater occipital nerve.

Therefore, greater occipital nerve blocks are not the singular test for cervicogenic headache. Other blocks would be required to establish a cervical source in those patients.

However, even the responses in those patients who obtained complete relief are difficult to interpret. There are no structures in the distribution of the greater occipital nerve that are known to be a source of chronic pain. Distal to the site at which it was blocked, the nerve supplies only the skin of the scalp and the occipitalis muscle. Ironically, it supplies no cervical structure. So, response to greater occipital nerve block is not evidence of a cervical source of pain and ironically, actually refutes a diagnosis of cervicogenic headache. The only sense of "cervical" is that the greater occipital nerve is a cervical nerve.

The physiological effect of greater occipital nerve blocks is not known. Animal studies have shown that stimulation of the greater occipital nerve facilitates responses in the trigeminocervical nucleus to noxious stimulation of the dura mater.[26] The converse effects of blocking the nerve on this interaction have not been studied, but the prospect applies that greater occipital nerve blocks might down-regulate non-specific headache mechanisms, and do not imply a cervical source of pain.

In another study, 14 patients underwent a variety of blocks of the greater occipital nerve, the C2, C3, C4, and C5 spinal nerves, and the C2–3 zygapophysial joint.[27] The spinal nerve blocks were performed without fluoroscopic control, so their accuracy is not known. Responses were assessed only at 20 minutes after the block. No control blocks were used.

One patient obtained complete relief of pain after both greater occipital nerve and C2 spinal nerve blocks, and one after C2 blocks only. One patient obtained complete relief after each of greater occipital, C2, and C5 blocks, and one after greater occipital, C2, and C4 blocks. Another had complete relief after greater occipital, C2 spinal nerve, and C2–3 joint blocks. One patient was relieved only by C2–3 joint blocks.

These results paint no consistent picture. Responses to blocks at multiple and displaced sites indicates either multiple sources for the same headache, or non-specific responses. Without controls, the latter cannot be excluded.

In accordance with the criteria proposed for cervical sources of headache (Box 23.2), it has been shown in normal volunteers and in patients that headache can be produced by noxious stimulation of the atlanto-occipital joints,[28] the lateral atlanto-axial joints,[28] the C2–3 zygapophysial joints,[29] and the C2–3 intervertebral disc.[30,31] Thus, for these structures, criterion 1 has been satisfied.

To various extents, these structures have been tested as sources of headache by anesthetizing them in patients presenting with headache. Diagnostic blocks of the cervical joints satisfy criteria 2 and 3 (Box 23.2). The C2–3 intervertebral disc has been excused, for there is no established means of reliably anesthetizing that structure. The multiple small nerves that innervate this disc cannot be discretely and specifically anesthetized.

Joint blocks require special facilities and special skills. In order to be accurate and safe, they must be performed under fluoroscopic guidance. Cervical joints can be anesthetized using either intra-articular injections (Figure 23.1) or blocks of the nerves that innervate the joint. The C2–3 zygapophysial joint is innervated by the third occipital nerve, and can be blocked by anesthetizing that nerve where it crosses the joint (Figure 23.2). Intra-articular blocks are rendered specific by injecting contrast medium to show that the block remains inside the target joint. Nerve blocks are rendered specific by using tiny volumes (0.3 ml) of local anesthetic.

Relief of headache following intra-articular injections of local anesthetic into the lateral atlanto-axial joint was initially reported in small case reports.[32,33,34] Later, a more extensive case series described complete relief of headache in 62% of 34 patients in whom lateral atlanto-axial joint blocks were performed.[35]

None of these studies incorporated any form of control block. Therefore, they do not provide incontrovertible evidence of headache stemming from the

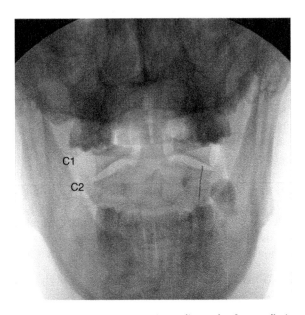

Figure 23.1. A postero-anterior radiograph of a needle in place in a right lateral atlanto-axial joint for the purpose of an intra-articular block.

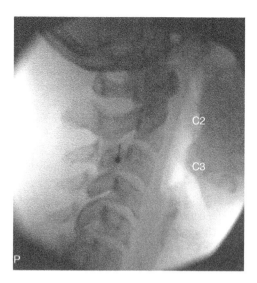

Figure 23-2. A lateral radiograph of the upper neck showing a needle in position to block the third occipital nerve where it crosses the C2–3 zygapophysial joint.

lateral atlanto-axial joints. Nevertheless, they do illustrate how blocks can be performed, and provide prima facie evidence that these joints appear to be the source of pain in some patients with headache.

More rigorous studies have investigated the C2–3 joint. They used double-blind, controlled blocks, under fluoroscopic guidance, using alternate agents: either a short-acting agent (lidocaine 2%) or a long-acting agent (bupivacaine 0.5%). The definition of a positive response was complete relief of pain, for the entire duration of action of the local anesthetic agent used.[36,37] In a series of 100 patients with neck pain after whiplash, 27% were relieved of their headache following these blocks.[36] Among those patients in whom headache was the dominant presenting symptom, 53% were relieved of their headache when the C2–3 joint was blocked. This study validated earlier reports of what had been described as third occipital headache, in uncontrolled descriptive studies.[38,39] A review paper reported that C2–3 is the most common zygapophysial joint responsible for headache, followed by C3–4. Only rarely are joints below C3–4 the source of headache.[37]

RESOLUTION

It is possible to reconcile the "clinical" and the "arthrological" approach to cervicogenic headache. Pivotal to this reconciliation is that the clinical approach must be tempered.

None of the clinical criteria for cervicogenic headache, alone or in combination, is perfectly valid. Clinical diagnosis will always overlap between cervicogenic headache, migraine, and tension-type headache;

and there is no evidence that the criteria for cervicogenic headache are valid for a cervical source of pain. However, the operational criteria of Antonaci et al.[16] (Box 23.1) provide for a tempered approach.

Cervicogenic headache can be suspected as a *possible* diagnosis in patients with pain that appears to start in the neck and spread to the head. This pattern of spread is consistent with the concept of cervicogenic headache being pain referred from the neck. In typical cases, the pain will be unilateral, but the pain can be bilateral if the patient has bilateral sources of pain in the neck. So, the liberalized version of the unilaterality criterion applies.[3,16]

Satisfying three additional criteria promotes the diagnosis form *possible* to *probable* cervicogenic headache. Some of these criteria, such as provocation of pain by neck movement, serve to implicate a cervical source of pain, but do not actually prove a cervical source. Others serve to exclude competing diagnoses. By definition, migraine is a periodic headache. A headache that is not periodic and is more continuous in character is less likely to be migraine and, ipso facto, is more likely to be cervicogenic. Similarly, migraine has associated features such as nausea, vomiting, and photophobia. The absence of these features renders migraine less likely and cervicogenic headache more probable.

The clinical approach, however, does not provide a definitive diagnosis. It provides no more than a suspicion or a probable diagnosis. Ultimately, the diagnosis rests on establishing a cervical source of pain.

Theoretically, a cervical source might be found by clinical examination but, to date, no clinical sign, or set of signs, has been shown to be both reliable and valid for any proven cervical source of pain. Nor has any imaging test been shown to be valid in the diagnosis of either neck pain or cervicogenic headache.

Diagnostic blocks are the only currently available means by which a cervical source of pain can be established. To be valid those blocks must be performed accurately and under controlled conditions.

These, in fact, have become the criteria for cervicogenic headache in the most recent taxonomy of the International Headache Society[40] (Box 23.3). Those criteria emphasize that the diagnosis cannot be made on clinical grounds. Controlled diagnostic blocks are required.

These criteria are probably culturally antithetical to most practitioners in the headache field, for they have been accustomed to making a diagnosis of other forms of headache largely from the history, and perhaps supplemented by a clinical examination. To say that this cannot be done for cervicogenic headache is tantamount to saying "you cannot make the diagnosis." For this reason, some, if not many practitioners decline to make the diagnosis, or even to entertain it.

BOX 23.3
DIAGNOSTIC CRITERIA FOR CERVICOGENIC HEADACHE, AS PROPOSED BY THE INTERNATIONAL HEADACHE SOCIETY[40]

Diagnostic criteria

A. Pain referred from a source in the neck and perceived in one or more regions of the head and/or face, fulfilling criteria C and D.

B. Clinical, laboratory and/or imaging evidence of a disorder or lesion within the cervical spine or soft tissues of the neck known to be, or generally accepted as, a valid cause of headache.[1]

C. Evidence that the pain can be attributed to the neck disorder or lesion based on at least one of the following:
   1. demonstration of clinical signs that implicate a source of pain in the neck[2]
   2. abolition of headache following diagnostic blockade of a cervical structure or its nerve supply using placebo or other adequate controls.[3]

D. Pain resolves within 3 months after successful treatment of the causative disorder or lesion.

Notes

1. Tumors, fractures, infections and rheumatoid arthritis of the upper cervical spine have not been validated formally as causes of headache, but are nevertheless accepted as valid causes when demonstrated to be so in individual cases. Cervical spondylosis and osteochondritis are NOT accepted as valid causes fulfilling criterion B. When myofascial tender spots are present, the headache should be coded under 2. *Tension-type headache*.

2. Clinical signs acceptable for criterion C1 must have demonstrated reliability and validity. The future task is the identification of such reliable and valid operational tests. Clinical features such as neck pain, focal neck tenderness, history of neck trauma, mechanical exacerbation of pain, unilaterality, coexisting shoulder pain, reduced range of motion in the neck, nuchal onset, nausea, vomiting, photophobia, etc. are not unique to cervicogenic headache. These may be features of cervicogenic headache, but they do not define relationship between the disorder and the source of the headache.

3. Abolition of headache means complete relief of headache, indicated by a score of zero on a visual analogue scale (VAS). Nevertheless, acceptable as fulfilling criterion C2 is ≥ 90% reduction in pain to a level of < 5 on a 100-point VAS.

Furthermore, the blocks required to make the diagnosis are not office procedures. Greater occipital nerve blocks are not the appropriate procedure. The necessary blocks target the joints of the cervical spine, and perhaps other structures such as intervertebral discs and spinal nerves. These blocks require advanced skills and special radiological facilities. Those requirements complicate the process of diagnosis, and constitute another reason why cervicogenic headache is not more widely entertained as a diagnosis. It is simply too difficult to make.

What should be recognized, however, is that none of these objections are scientific. There are firm data on the mechanism, sources, and causes of cervicogenic headache[41] (Chapter 22). Techniques for the blocks have been described.[42,43] The condition is common, particularly in patients with a history of trauma, among whom the prevalence is at least 53%.[41] Declining to pursue the diagnosis is a social decision. That decision, however, denies patients the opportunity for a valid diagnosis being made.

References

1. Fredriksen TA, Hovdal H, Sjaastad O. "Cervicogenic headache": clinical manifestation. Cephalalgia 1987; 7: 147–160.

2. Sjaastad O, Fredriksen TA, Pfaffenrath V. Cervicogenic headache: diagnostic criteria. Headache 1990; 30: 725–726.

3. Sjaastad O, Fredriksen TA, Pfaffenrath V. Cervicogenic headache: diagnostic criteria. Headache 1998; 38: 442–445.

4. Leone M, D'Amico D, Frediani F, Torri W, Sjaastad O, Bussone G. Clinical considerations on side-locked unilaterality in long-lasting primary headaches. Headache 1993; 33: 381–384.

5. D'Amico D, Leone M, Bussone G. Side-locked unilaterality and pain localization in long-lasting headaches: migraine, tension-type headache, and cervicogenic headache. Headache 1994; 34: 526–530.

6. Leone M, D'Amico D, Moschiano F, Frainotti M, Filippini G, Bussone G. Possible identification of cervicogenic headache amongst patients with migraine: an analysis of 374 headaches. Headache 1995; 35: 461–464.

7. Leone M, D'Amico D, Grazzi L, Attanasio A, Bussone G. Cervicogenic headache: a critical review of the current diagnostic criteria. Pain 1998; 78: 1–5.

8. Bovim G. Cervicogenic headache, migraine, and tension-type headache: pressure-pain threshold measurements. Pain 1992; 51: 169–173.

9. Jull G, Barrett C, Magee R, Ho P. Further clinical clarification of the muscle dysfunction in cervical headache. Cephalalgia 1999; 19: 179–185.

10. Fredriksen TA, Fougner R, Tengerund A, Sjaastad O. Cervicogenic headache: radiological investigations concerning head/neck. Cephalalgia 1989; 9: 139–146.

11. Pfaffenrath V, Dandekar R, Pollman W. Cervicogenic headache: the clinical picture, radiological findings and hypotheses on its pathophysiology. Headache 1987; 27: 495–499.

12. Zwart JA. Neck mobility in different headache disorders. Headache 1997; 37: 6–11.

13. van Suijlekom JA, de Vet HCW, van den Berg SGM, Weber WEJ. Interobserver reliability of diagnostic criteria for cervicogenic headache. Cephalalgia 1999; 19: 817–823.

14. van Suijlekom HA, de Vet HCW, van den Berg SGM, Weber WEJ. Interobserver reliability in physical examination of the cervical spine in patients with headache. Headache 2000; 40: 581–586.

15. Vincent M. Validation of criteria for cervicogenic headache. Functional Neurology 1998; 13: 74–75.

16. Antonaci F, Ghirmai S, Bono S, Sandrini G, Nappi G. Cervicogenic headache: evaluation of the original diagnostic criteria. Cephalalgia 2001; 21: 573–583.

17. Headache Classification Committee of the International Headache Society. Classification and diagnostic criteria for headache disorders, cranial neuralgias and facial pain. Cephalalgia 1988; 8: 1–96.

18. Jull G, Bogduk N, Marsland A. The accuracy of manual diagnosis for cervical zygapophysial joint pain syndromes. Med J Aust 1988; 148: 233–236.

19. Fjellner A, Bexander C, Faleij R, Strender LE. Interexaminer reliability in physical examination of the cervical spine. J Manip Physiol Ther 1999; 22: 511–516.

20. Smedmark V, Wallin M, Arvidsson I. Inter-examiner reliability in assessing passive intervertebral motion of the cervical spine. Man Ther 2000; 5: 97–101.

21. Jull G, Zito G, Trott P, Potter H, Shirley D, Richardson C. Inter-examiner reliability to detect painful upper cervical joint dysfunction. Aust J Physio 1997; 43: 125–129.

22. Bogduk N. Four times tables. Aust J Physio 1997; 43: 290–291.

23. Jull G. Author's response. Aust J Physio 1997; 43: 292.

24. Bogduk N. Headaches and the cervical spine. An editorial. Cephalalgia 1984; 4: 7–8.

25. Bovim G, Sand T. Cervicogenic headache, migraine without aura and tension-type headache: diagnostic blockade of greater occipital and supra-orbital nerves. Pain 1992; 51: 43–48.

26. Bartsch T, Goadsby PJ. Stimulation of the greater occipital nerve induces increased central excitability of dural afferent input. Brain 2002; 125: 1496–1509.

27. Bovim G, Berg R, Dale LG. Cervicogenic headache: anaesthetic blockades of cervical nerves (C2–C5) and facet joint (C2/C3). Pain 1992; 49: 315–320.

28. Dreyfuss P, Michaelsen M, Fletcher D. Atlanto-occipital and lateral atlanto-axial joint pain patterns. Spine 1994; 19: 1125–1131.

29. Dwyer A, Aprill C, Bogduk N. Cervical zygapophysial joint pain patterns. I. A study in normal volunteers. Spine 1990; 15: 453–457.

30. Schellhas KP, Smith MD, Gundry CR, Pollei SR. Cervical discogenic pain: prospective correlation of magnetic resonance imaging and discography in asymptomatic subjects and pain sufferers. Spine 1996; 21: 300–312.

31. Grubb SA, Kelly CK. Cervical discography: clinical implications from 12 years of experience. Spine 2000; 25: 1382–1389.

32. Ehni G, Benner B. Occipital neuralgia and the C1–2 arthrosis syndrome. J Neurosurg 1984; 61: 961–965.

33. Busch E, Wilson PR. Atlanto-occipital and atlanto-axial injections in the treatment of headache and neck pain. Reg Anesth 1989; 14(Suppl. 2): 45.

34. McCormick CC. Arthrography of the atlanto-axial (C1–C2) joints: technique and results. J Intervent Radiol 1987; 2: 9–13.

35. Aprill C, Axinn MJ, Bogduk N. Occipital headaches stemming from the lateral atlanto-axial (C1–2) joint. Cephalalgia 2002; 22: 15–22.

36. Lord S, Barnsley L, Wallis B, Bogduk N. Third occipital headache: a prevalence study. J Neurol Neurosurg Psychiat 1994; 57: 1187–1190.

37. Lord SM, Bogduk N. The cervical synovial joints as sources of post-traumatic headache. J Musculoskelet Pain 1996; 4: 81–94.

38. Bogduk N, Marsland A. On the concept of third occipital headache. J Neurol Neurosurg Psychiat 1986; 49: 775–780.

39. Bogduk N, Marsland A. The cervical zygapophysial joints as a source of neck pain. Spine 1988; 13: 610–617.

40. International Headache Society. The International Classification of Headache Disorders, 2nd edn. Cephalalgia 2004; 24 (Suppl. 1): 115–116.

41. Bogduk N. The neck and headaches. Neurol Clin N Am 2004; 22: 151–171.

42. International Spine Intervention Society. Lateral atlanto-axial joint blocks. In: Bogduk N (ed). Practice Guidelines for Spinal Diagnostic and Treatment Procedures. International Spine Intervention Society, San Francisco, 2004.

43. International Spine Intervention Society. Cervical medial branch blocks. In: Bogduk N (ed). Practice Guidelines for Spinal Diagnostic and Treatment Procedures. International Spine Intervention Society, San Francisco, 2004.

Cervicogenic headache: treatment

> **KEY POINTS**
>
> - Few treatments have been validated for cervicogenic headache.
>
> - For *probable* cervicogenic headache, exercises and gentle mobilization are the most pragmatic therapeutic option.
>
> - If the source of pain can be traced to a particular joint, intra-articular injections of steroids might be entertained.
>
> - For third occipital headache, radiofrequency neurotomy is the only treatment shown to provide complete relief of pain.
>
> - For pain from the lateral atlanto-axial joints, arthrodesis may be an option.
>
> - The treatment of occipital neuralgia by injections or neurectomy has not been shown to provide lasting relief of pain.

Despite the longstanding interest in headaches of cervical origin, the literature provides little evidence concerning their treatment. For rare and unusual causes, standard surgical interventions are both available and appropriate: aneurysms can be clipped or repaired; tumors of the posterior cranial fossa can be excised; subluxation of the atlas due to rheumatoid arthritis can be treated by arthrodesis. For the majority of common causes, however, a proven treatment has not been established.

Trigger points

The treatment of trigger points with injections of local anesthetic has not been subjected to any form of scientific study. Indeed, a systematic review found no evidence that needling therapies have any efficacy beyond that of placebo.[1]

Manual therapy

Various forms of physical and manual therapy have been advocated for headaches believed to be of cervical origin. Most of the literature, however, consists of case reports or case series.[2] The few randomized controlled studies provided follow-up of only 1 or 3 weeks,[3,4,5] and provided conflicting results.[2]

The largest and most recent study provided encouraging results.[6] It showed that treatment with manual therapy, specific exercises, or manual therapy plus exercises was significantly more effective at reducing headache frequency and intensity than was no specific care by a general practitioner. Manual therapy alone, however, was not more effective than exercises alone, and combining the two interventions did not achieve better outcomes. Some 76% of patients achieved greater than 50% reduction in headache frequency at the 7-week follow-up, and 35% achieved complete relief. At 12 months, 72% had greater than 50% reduction in headache frequency, but the proportion that had complete relief was not reported. Corresponding figures for reduction in pain intensity were not reported.

C2 neuralgia

There is no evidence that C2 neuralgia responds to pharmacotherapy.[7] Surgery appears to be the only definitive means of treatment. Nerves entrapped by scar can be liberated;[8] meningiomas can be excised.[9] With respect to venous anomalies, resection of the vascular abnormality alone does not reliably relieve the pain; resection or thermocoagulation of the nerve appears to be necessary to guarantee relief of pain.[7] This calls into question whether the vascular anomaly is really the responsible lesion, particularly in view of the fact that in 50% of cadavers the C2 roots are surrounded by a dense venous network.[10]

A study described the result of C2 ganglionectomy, not expressly for patients with C2 neuralgia but for patients with occipital pain.[11] Nineteen of 39 patients (49%) obtained greater than 90% relief of their pain. However, outcomes were better in certain subgroups. A successful outcome was achieved in 64% of 22 patients with a history of trauma, and in 78% of 23 patients with shooting, stabbing, or burning pain. These latter patients would seem to correspond to those with C2 neuralgia described in other studies.

Occipital neuralgia

Since it was first described, occipital neuralgia has attracted a variety of surgical interventions. These include "liberation" of the greater occipital nerve, greater occipital neurectomy, and transection of the roots of that nerve.

Liberation of the greater occipital nerve is based on the presumption that, somehow, it has become trapped by scar tissue or other abnormalities at the point where it leaves the posterior neck muscles to become cutaneous. The treatment is directed at removing the offending material from the vicinity of the nerve. There are few reports of the efficacy of this operation. The most detailed study reported that liberation of the nerve initially relieves headache in some 80% of cases, but the relief has a median duration of only some 3–6 months.[12]

Greater occipital neurectomy requires transecting the greater occipital where it leaves the posterior neck muscles, with or without avulsing it. This procedure was advocated by Hunter and Mayfield[13] in their original description of occipital neuralgia, and was subsequently endorsed by others.[14] For some 30 years, it remained a standard procedure for occipital neuralgia. However, because it is a radical, if not brutal, procedure, it eventually attracted criticism.[15] Not only did greater occipital neurectomy lack an etiology that logically justified excision, let alone avulsion, of the nerve, the efficacy of the procedure was never established. The only study that provides quantitative data reported that excision of the greater occipital nerve provides relief in some 70% of patients, but this relief has a median duration of only 244 days.[16] Since the nerve has been excised, relief cannot be reinstated by repeating the procedure.

Some surgeons extended the concept of greater occipital neurectomy by targeting the dorsal roots that subtend this nerve.[17,18] Dorsal rhizotomy at C1–3 or C1–4 has provided some patients with complete relief for 1–4 years, but some patients nevertheless suffer recurrences.[19] Partial posterior rhizotomy at C1–3 appears to achieve good relief while preserving touch sensation; but not all patients respond adequately.[20] Unfortunately, these procedures are so radical that they provide us with little insight into the mechanisms of occipital neuralgia, save to warn that even complete deafferentation of the affected region does not guarantee relief of pain.

Neck tongue syndrome

Data on the treatment of neck tongue syndrome are limited to case reports. Some investigators have found immobilization by a soft collar to be adequate therapy;[21,22] others have used spinal manipulation.[23] Some have resorted to atlanto-axial fusion[24] or resection of the C2 spinal nerves.[25] Operative findings have confirmed that the syndrome involves compression of the C2 spinal nerves by the lateral atlanto-axial joint.[25] These case reports provide a list of options for neck tongue syndrome, but neither individually nor collectively do they provide evidence of a proven treatment for this condition.

Lateral atlanto-axial joint pain

Techniques have only recently been developed for the diagnosis of cervicogenic headache specifically stemming from the lateral atlanto-axial joint. These techniques have not been adopted into common practice. Consequently, there has been little opportunity to evaluate conservative treatments for this condition. The efficacy of exercises or manual therapy is unknown.

Some practitioners use periarticular[26] or intra-articular[27] injections of corticosteroids, in the hope that these might provide some degree of lasting relief, but no data are available on the effect of such injections, either in the short term or the long term. The only treatment whose long-term outcome has been described is arthrodesis of the atlas. In a small number of cases, fusion has been reported as producing complete and lasting relief of pain.[28,29]

Nonspecific cervicogenic headache

Most studies that have explored treatment for cervicogenic headache did not specify the source of pain. They selected their patients on the basis of clinical criteria only (Chapter 23).

In one study, injections of corticosteroids onto the nerve were used to treat cervicogenic headache.[30] Of 180 patients with cervicogenic headache, 169 obtained relief from the injection of 160 mg of depot methylprednisolone onto the nerve, but the relief lasted only between 10 and 77 days. Thus, steroid injections may be temporarily palliative, but they do not constitute definitive treatment.

Other studies have pursued more invasive interventions. In one study, patients were selected for surgery if they satisfied the clinical criteria for cervicogenic headache and obtained relief of headache from diagnostic blockade of the C2 spinal nerve.[31] They underwent decompression and microsurgical neurolysis of the C2 spinal nerve, with excision of scar, and ligamentous and vascular elements that compressed the nerve. Fourteen of 31 patients were rendered pain-free. Details on the remaining patients are incomplete but ostensibly 51% gained what was called "adequate" relief, and 11% suffered a recurrence. The data presented do not reliably indicate how enduring these outcomes are. Those patients who were rendered pain-free were followed for 16 ± 21 months (mean $\pm$ sd), which indicates a very wide range. For those with adequate relief the follow-up was 21 ± 18 months.

Another study purported to show that radiofrequency neurotomy of the cervical zygapophysial joints could be successful.[32] In this study, however, diagnostic blocks were expressly not performed to select a target level, and denervation was performed at all levels from C3 to C6. Even so, only one of 15 patients achieved complete relief of pain. A further 11 patients were described as having good relief of pain but this outcome was not defined.

A randomized, placebo-controlled study of radiofrequency neurotomy showed no benefit for patients with cervicogenic headache diagnosed on the basis of clinical features.[33] This outcome underscores the lack of validity of clinical diagnosis for this condition, and highlights the importance of achieving complete relief of pain from controlled diagnostic blocks as the indication for radiofrequency neurotomy.[34]

Discogenic pain

The only available treatment for cervical discogenic pain is arthrodesis of the responsible segment. For the treatment of cervicogenic headache, arthrodesis has not been systematically studied. One descriptive study reports encouraging results.[35] It described nine patients in whom discography at C2–3 reproduced their headache. Four of these patients obtained complete relief of their headache, at a minimum follow-up of 24 months. An additional two patients obtained greater than 50% relief of their pain.

Third occipital headache

No form of pharmacological or physical therapy has ever been tested for this type of headache, and none has been proposed to work. The only available treatments are invasive in nature.

Third occipital headache is amenable to treatment with intra-articular injections of steroids, but the efficacy of this intervention has been reported only in one descriptive study.[36] At 19 months following such injections, 11% of patients were free of pain. A further 50% had a reduced frequency of headaches. That study, however, was not controlled. Consequently it is not evident if it is the administration of steroids or simply the act of injection into the joint that is the active component of the therapeutic effect. Nevertheless, intra-articular injection would seem to be a safe and expedient intervention that could benefit some patients.

The only other known treatment for third occipital headache is radiofrequency neurotomy. This procedure involves denervating the C2–3 zygapophysial joint percutaneously by placing an electrode parallel to the nerve where it crosses the joint (Figure 24.1) and using it to coagulate the nerve. To be effective, the essential indication for the procedure is complete relief of pain following controlled, diagnostic blocks of the third occipital nerve.

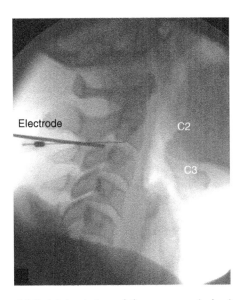

Figure 24.1 A lateral view of the upper cervical spine showing an electrode in place for radiofrequency neurotomy of the third occipital nerve where it crosses the C2–3 zygapophysial joint.

When first evaluated, radiofrequency neurotomy of the third occipital nerve did not reliably achieve relief of pain.[37] The authors warned that radiofrequency neurotomy should not be adopted until technical deficiencies of the procedure had been overcome. That has now been achieved.

Several technical requirements were necessary to ensure the efficacy of third occipital neurotomy.[38] The electrode must be in place during coagulation, lest it becomes dislodged from the target nerve during the procedure; and multiple lesions must be made in order to encompass all possible locations of the nerve. Since the electrode makes only a small lesion, it is critical that electrodes be placed no further than one electrode-width apart. If that criterion is not satisfied, the nerve may escape coagulation between electrode placements. The procedure is described in detail in the practice guidelines of the International Spine Intervention Society.[39]

A study using the revised technique showed that complete relief of pain could be achieved in 88% of patients. The median duration of relief was 297 days with 13 of the 49 patients still having continuing relief at the time of review. For patients in whom headaches recurred, relief could be reinstated by repeating the neurotomy. By repeating neurotomy as required, some patients have been able to maintain relief of their headache for longer than 2 years.

Although radiofrequency neurotomy for third occipital headache has not been subjected to a controlled trial, the procedure has otherwise been tested in patients with neck pain. A randomized, placebo-controlled trial showed that responses to radiofrequency neurotomy are not due to placebo effects.[40] Its success in the treatment of third occipital headache, therefore, cannot be dismissed as a placebo effect.

RECOMMENDATIONS

For patients with a clinical diagnosis of *probable* cervicogenic headache (Chapter 23), it would seem reasonable to undertake treatment with exercises and manual therapy in the form of passive cervical mobilization.[6] In that regard, it should be recognized that manual therapy is not synonymous with manipulative. There is no evidence that forceful, or high-velocity manipulation is either safe or effective for cervicogenic headache. Any manual therapy should be limited to gentle, oscillatory movements of the upper cervical joints.

For patients who do not respond to this conservative intervention, investigations can be undertaken to establish the source of pain, if possible. Discography or blocks of the upper cervical joints can be performed.

For discogenic pain, arthrodesis of the C2–3 segment appears to be an effective option.[35] There are no known alternatives for discogenic pain.

If the lateral atlanto-axial joint proves to be the source, there is no proven treatment. This should be explained to the patient. Under those conditions, and with the informed consent of the patient, an intra-articular injection of corticosteroid might be ventured. Practitioners wishing to pursue this treatment should determine what the regulatory and ethical restrictions might be in their geographic area of practice. Some jurisdictions might require approval from an ethics committee before a treatment is undertaken, for which there are no published data of efficacy, and which might be considered experimental.

If the C2–3 zygapophysial joint proves to be the source of pain, two options are available. A small proportion of patients might benefit from an intra-articular injection of corticosteroid.[36] Otherwise, third occipital neurotomy is an established option.[38] The critical indication for that procedure, however, is that the patient must have obtained complete relief of their headache following controlled, diagnostic blocks of the third occipital nerve. There is explicit evidence that neurotomy does not work if this criterion has not been satisfied.

References

1. Cummings TM, White AR. Needling therapies in the management of myofascial trigger point pain: a systematic review. Arch Phys Med Rehabil 2001; 82: 986–992.
2. Haldeman S, Dagenais S. Cervicogenic headaches: a critical review. Spine J 2001; 1: 31–46.
3. Nilsson N. A randomized controlled trial of the effect of spinal manipulation in the treatment of cervicogenic headache. J Manipul Physiol Ther 1995; 18: 435–440.
4. Nilsson N, Christensen HW, Hartvigsen J. The effect of spinal manipulation in the treatment of cervicogenic headache. J Manipul Physiol Ther 1997; 20: 326–330.
5. Vernon HT. Spinal manipulation and headaches of cervical origin. J Manipul Physiol Ther 1989; 12: 455–468.
6. Jull G, Trott P, Potter H, Zito G, et al. A randomized controlled trial of exercise and manipulative therapy for cervicogenic headache. Spine 2002; 27: 1835–1843.
7. Jansen J, Bardosi A, Hildebrandt J, Lucke A. Cervicogenic, hemicranial attacks associated with vascular irritation or compression of the cervical nerve root C2: clinical manifestations and morphological findings. Pain 1989; 39: 203–212.
8. Poletti CE, Sweet WH. Entrapment of the C2 root and ganglion by the atlanto-epistrophic ligament: clinical syndrome and surgical anatomy. Neurosurgery 1990; 27: 288–291.
9. Kurltzky, A. Cluster headache-like pain caused by an upper cervical meningioma. Cephalalgia 1984; 4: 185–186.
10. Bovim G, Bonamico L, Fredriksen TA, Lindboe C, Stolt-Nielsen A, Sjaastad O. Topographic variations in the peripheral course of the greater occipital nerve. Spine 1991; 16: 475–478.
11. Lozano A, Vanderlinden G, Bachoo R, Rothbart P. Microsurgical C-2 ganglionectomy for chronic intractable occipital pain. J Neurosurg 1998; 89: 359–365.
12. Bovim G, Fredriksen TA, Stolt-Nielsen A, Sjaastad O. Neurolysis of the greater occipital nerve in cervicogenic headache: a follow up study. Headache 1992; 32: 175–179.
13. Hunter CR, Mayfield FH. Role of the upper cervical roots in the production of pain in the head. Am J Surg 1949; 78: 743–749.
14. Murphy JP. Occipital neurectomy in the treatment of headache. Maryland State Med J 1969; 18: 62–66.
15. Weinberger LM. Cervico-occipital pain and its surgical treatment: the myth of the bony millstones. Am J Surg 1978; 135: 243–247.
16. Anthony M. Headache and the greater occipital nerve. Clin Neurol Neurosurg 1992; 94: 297–301.
17. Chambers WR. Posterior rhizotomy of the second and third cervical nerves for occipital pain. JAMA 1954; 155: 431–432.
18. Cusson D, King A. Cervical rhizotomy in the management of some cases of occipital neuralgia. Guthrie Clin Bull 1960; 29: 198–208.
19. Horowitz MB, Yonas H. Occipital neuralgia treated by intradural dorsal nerve root sectioning. Cephalalgia 1993; 13: 354–360.
20. Dubuisson D. Treatment of occipital neuralgia by partial posterior rhizotomy at C1–3. J Neurosurg 1995; 82: 581–586.
21. Fortin C J, Biller J. Neck tongue syndrome. Headache 1985; 25: 255–258.
22. Cassidy JD, Diakow PRP, de Korompay VL, Munkacsi I, Yong-Hing K. Treatment of neck-tongue syndrome by spinal manipulation: a report of three cases. Pain Clinic 986; 1: 41–46.
23. Webb J, March L, Tyndall A. The neck-tongue syndrome: occurrence with cervical arthritis as well as normals. J Rheumatol 1984; 11: 530–533.
24. Bertoft ES, Westerberg CE. Further observations on the neck-tongue syndrome. Cephalalgia 1985; 5(Suppl. 3): 312–313.
25. Elisevich K, Stratford J, Bray G, Finlayson M. Neck tongue syndrome: operative management. J Neurol Neurosurg Psychiatry 1984; 47: 407–409.
26. Ehni G, Benner B. Occipital neuralgia and the C1–2 arthrosis syndrome. J Neurosurg 1984; 61: 961–965.
27. Aprill C, Axinn MJ, Bogduk N. Occipital headaches stemming from the lateral atlanto-axial (C1–2) joint. Cephalalgia 2002; 22: 15–22.
28. Joseph B, Kumar B. Gallie's fusion for atlantoaxial arthrosis with occipital neuralgia. Spine 1994; 19: 454–455.
29. Ghanayem AJ, Leventhal M, Bohlman HH. Osteoarthrosis of the atlanto-axial joints: long-term follow-up after treatment with arthrodesis. J Bone Joint Surg 1996; 78A: 1300–1307.
30. Anthony M. Cervicogenic headache: prevalence and response to local steroid therapy. Clin Exp Rheumatol 2000; 18(Suppl. 19): S59–S64.
31. Pikus HJ, Phillips JM. Characteristics of patients successfully treated for cervicogenic headache by surgical decompression of the second cervical root. Headache 1995; 35: 621–629.
32. van Suijlekom HA, van Kleef M, Barendse GAM, Sluijter ME, Sjaastad O, Weber WEJ. Radiofrequency cervical zygapophyseal joint neurotomy for cervicogenic headaches: a prospective study of 15 patients. Funct Neurol 1998; 13: 297–303.
33. Stovner LJ, Kolstad F, Helde G. Radiofrequency denervation of facet joints C2-C6 in cervicogenic headache: a randomized, double-blind, sham-controlled study. Cephalalgia 2004; 24: 821–830.
34. Bogduk N. Editorial. Cephalalgia 2004; 24: 819–820.

35. Schofferman J, Garges K, Goldthwaite N, Koestler M, Libby E. Upper cervical anterior diskectomy and fusion improves discogenic cervical headaches. Spine 2002; 27: 2240–2244.

36. Slipman CW, Lipetz JS, Plastara CT, Jackson HW, Yang ST, Meyer AM. Therapeutic zygapophyseal joint injections for headache emanating from the C2–3 joint. Am J Phys Med Rehabil 2001; 80: 182–188.

37. Lord SM, Barnsley L, Bogduk N. Percutaneous radiofrequency neurotomy in the treatment of cervical zygapophysial joint pain: a caution. Neurosurgery 1995; 36: 732–739.

38. Govind J, King W, Bailey B, Bogduk N. Radiofrequency neurotomy for the treatment of third occipital headache. J Neurol Neurosurg Psychiatry 2003; 74: 88–93.

39. International Spine Intervention Society. Percutaneous radiofrequency cervical medial branch neurotomy. In: Bogduk N (ed). Practice Guidelines for Spinal Diagnostic and Treatment Procedures. International Spine Intervention Society, San Francisco, 2004: 249–284.

40. Lord SM, Barnsley L, Wallis BJ, McDonald GJ, Bogduk N. Percutaneous radio-frequency neurotomy for chronic cervical zygapophysial-joint pain. N Engl J Med 1996; 335: 1721–1726.

6 Statistical terms

Statistical terms

Statistics can be used to determine and describe how well a device works. In clinical practice, that device may be a diagnostic test or a treatment. Different statistics apply to diagnostic tests and to treatments, but they each have in common the objective of expressing, in a single number, just how well the test or treatment works. This final chapter provides a short explanation of terms used in this text in the evaluation of various diagnostic tests and treatments used for neck pain.

CONFIDENCE INTERVALS

Sometimes, investigators report observations or results in the form of a proportion or a percentage. For example, they might report that 20 out of 25 patients (80%) exhibited a particular clinical sign; or they might conclude that, since 30 out of 40 patients responded to a treatment, the success rate was 75%. Those proportions are reported as figures indicative of what readers should expect to encounter were they to adopt or follow the author's methods. This is not entirely correct.

When investigators conduct a study, they use a sample of patients. The conclusions that they draw are based on the behavior of that sample. However, observations made in that sample are not necessarily what others will experience if they study another sample. Different samples may exhibit different responses. Proportions observed in one sample may not be encountered in another.

Any proportion is not an exact figure. It is accompanied by an error-range, which is dependent on the size of the sample.

A convenient manner in which to represent this error range is the 95% confidence interval (CI) of a proportion. Mathematically, this range is given by the formula:

$$p^* = p \pm 1.96 \sqrt{\frac{p(1-p)}{n}}$$

where p is the observed proportion in a sample of n subjects, and p^* is the 95% confidence interval of that proportion.

The 95% confidence interval is the range of values of p that others might expect to encounter in 95% of all repetitions of the same study. That range is critically dependent on the sample size.

For example, if an investigator obtains a success rate of 8 out of 10, that does not mean that others should also expect an 80% success rate. The 95% confidence interval for 8 out of 10 is obtained from:

$$p^* = 0.8 \pm 1.96\sqrt{\frac{0.8(1-0.8)}{10}}$$

$$p^* = 0.8 \pm 0.25$$

This means that other observers have a 95% chance of encountering a success rate anywhere from as low as 55% to as high as 100%.

If the original report had been obtained in a larger sample, e.g. 50, the expected success rate is still not 80%, but is substantially closer, i.e.:

$$p^* = 0.8 \pm 1.96\sqrt{\frac{0.8(1-0.8)}{50}}$$

$$p^* = 0.8 \pm 0.11$$

In this case, someone who repeated the study would have a 95% chance of encountering a success rate anywhere from as low as 69% to as high as 91%.

These remarks are not restricted to investigators who undertake scientific studies. Whenever any practitioner adopts a test or a treatment and applies it to their own patients, they are effectively reproducing the experiment. They should not expect to encounter the same results as those reported in the literature. What they should expect, in their own hands, is a result somewhere in the 95% confidence interval of the reported result. This may the same as the originally reported result, or it may be better or worse.

Reporting the 95% confidence interval of a proportion gives practitioners a realistic idea of what to expect. If authors do not provide those confidence intervals, readers can calculate them for themselves, using the formula provided above.

DIAGNOSTIC TESTS

There are two separate determinants of how well a diagnostic test works. One is *reliability*. The other is *validity*. For a diagnostic test to be held to "work," it must be both reliable and valid. Conversely, the test cannot work if it lacks either reliability or validity.

Reliability

Reliability is the extent to which two observers obtain the same results when using the same diagnostic test on the same sample of patients. It is determined by having two observers independently apply the test on the same patients, and recording the results in a contingency table (Table 25.1).

In such a table, the total number (N) of patients in the sample is $a + b + c + d$; a constitutes the number of patients in whom both observers found that the test was positive; d is the number of patients in whom both observers found that the tests was negative; b is the number of patients in whom observer number one found the test to be positive but observer number two found it to be negative; and c is the number of patients in whom observer number one found the test to be negative but observer number two found it to be positive. Such a table shows that the observers agreed that the test was positive in a cases, and agreed that the test was negative in d cases. Their apparent rate of agreement is $[(a + d)/N] \times 100\%$.

The apparent rate of agreement, however, is not an accurate measure of how good the test is, for it incorporates agreement that might have occurred by chance alone. The true agreement is provided by discounting the apparent agreement for agreement by chance. This is illustrated in Figure 25.1, which shows that if there is not complete agreement in all cases, the observed agreement (P_o) is less than complete agreement by the extent to which there is disagreement. The figure also illustrates that complete agreement consists of two, hypothetical, parts: the agreement expected by chance alone (P_e) and the range available for possible agreement beyond chance alone ($1-P_e$).

The observed agreement consists one portion due to agreement by chance alone, and another portion that is the agreement beyond chance alone (P_o-P_e). In determining the reliability of the test, credit is not given to the observers for that agreement which they achieved by chance alone. Their true skill, and the strength of

Table 25.1 A contingency table from which the reliability of a diagnostic test can be derived

Observer one	Observer two	
	Positive	Negative
Positive	a	b
Negative	c	d

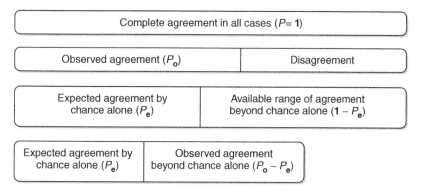

Figure 25.1 The distinction between observed agreement and agreement beyond chance.

the test, is determined by how well they agreed beyond chance alone.

That is established by measuring how far their observed agreement extends into the range of agreement available beyond chance alone, and is expressed by a statistic called *kappa*, where:

$$kappa = (P_o - P_e)/(1 - P_e).$$

In words, kappa is the extent to which the observed agreement (discounted for chance) fills the range of possible agreement available (also discounted for chance).

An example to help understand this concept is a multiple choice examination. If there are 100 questions, each with four choices, a candidate could, on average, answer one in four questions correctly simply by guessing. By chance alone they could score 25%. A candidate who scores 65% has not demonstrated a proficiency of 65%, since 25 of those 65 marks could have been gained by chance alone. Their true skill is demonstrated by how well they performed beyond chance alone. Accordingly their raw score (65) is discounted by the number of questions that they could have answered correctly by chance alone (25), which yields 40. Similarly, the total number of questions (100) is discounted by the number of questions that might have been answered correctly by chance alone (25) to yield the available number of questions that might have been answered correctly beyond chance alone (75). The true skill of the candidate then is the proportion of the available number of questions (75) that the candidate correctly answered (40), i.e. 40/75 = 53%. The true skill of the candidate, discounted for chance, is 53%, not the raw score of 65%.

Not obvious in the determination of reliability is how the expected agreement by chance alone should be estimated. This is based on what the two observers find, on average, which is shown by the sums of the columns and rows of the contingency table (Table 25.2).

This table shows that, overall, observer one recorded positive findings in $(a + b)$ cases. The proportion of cases that this observer found to be positive is $(a + b)/N$. On average, therefore, this observer would record positive findings in $(a + b)/N$ of all cases presented. Meanwhile, observer two found $(a + c)$ cases to be positive. If these cases were presented to observer one, the number that would be expected to be recorded as positive by chance alone would be $(a + c) \times (a + b)/N$.

Similarly, the proportion of cases that observer one recorded as negative is $(c + d)/N$. The number of cases that observer two found to be negative is $(b + d)$. If these cases were presented to observer one, the number that would be expected to be recorded as negative by chance alone would be $(b + d) \times (c + d)/N$.

These derived numbers provide an estimate of the agreement expected by chance alone (P_e), i.e.

$$P_e = [(a + c)(a + b)/N + (b + d)(c + d)/N]/N$$

which is different from the observed agreement (P_o), viz.

$$P_o = (a + d)/N$$

Table 25.2 A contingency table from which agreement can be derived

Observer one	Observer two		
	Positive	*Negative*	*Totals*
Positive	a	b	a + b
Negative	c	d	c + d
Totals	a + c	b + d	N = a + b + c + d

From these equations, P_o, P_e, $(P_o–P_e)$, and $(1–P_e)$ can be calculated, and hence, kappa can be calculated. Readers interested in further reading about kappa can consult the original literature[1] or various other educational resources.[2,3]

For practical purposes, however, readers should understand that once calculated, kappa can range in value from 0 to 1, or from 0 to −1. Negative values of kappa indicate abject disagreement, which occurs only for very unreliable tests. For most tests, the values are positive. A value of 0 indicates no agreement beyond chance alone. A value of 1 indicates complete (i.e. perfect) agreement.

Values between 0 and 1 can be accorded a range of verbal descriptors (Table 25.3). The kappa values indicate quantitatively, and the descriptors indicate qualitatively, just how reliable the diagnostic test is.

If practitioners use diagnostic tests with high kappa scores, they can be confident that the reliability of the test is good. However, if the kappa score is low, practitioners should realize that the diagnostic test does not work well; that someone else using the same test on the same patient is not likely to obtain the same result. Consequently, there are grounds to question or to doubt the result that they have obtained.

The kappa score does not, and cannot, determine which of two observers is correct. It measures only how consistent any two observers are or might expect to be. But if consistency is lacking, the test—or how it is used— is defective. In essence, diagnostic tests with low kappa scores just do not work well enough to be reliable. Their results are little better than guessing, and do not reflect professional proficiency.

Validity

Validity is the measure of how well a diagnostic test actually establishes both the presence and the absence of a condition that it is intended to detect. It is determined by comparing the results of the diagnostic test with those of another test—called the criterion standard—which provides more direct evidence of the presence and absence of the condition. For diagnostic tests based on physical examination the criterion standard could be the result of X-ray examination, surgical findings, or post-mortem findings.

The numerical properties of a diagnostic test can be derived by constructing a contingency table, in which the results of a diagnostic test are compared with the results of the criterion standard when both are applied to the same sample of patients (Table 25.4). Two fundamental statistics can be derived from the columns of such a table.

The *sensitivity* of the test measures how well the test correctly detects positive cases. It is also known as the *true-positive rate*. It is calculated as $a/(a + c)$, where $(a + c)$ is the number of cases that truly have the condition, and a is the number of these cases that the test correctly detects. By inference, c is the number of cases with the condition that the test failed to detect.

The *specificity* of the test measures how well the test correctly detects the absence of the condition. It is also known as the *true-negative rate*. It is calculated as $d/(b + d)$, where $(b + d)$ is the number of cases that truly do not have the condition, and d is the number of these cases that the test correctly detects. By inference, b is the number of cases without the condition that the test failed to detect correctly, and which the test incorrectly found to be positive instead of negative. Accordingly, the ratio $b/(b + d)$ is the *false-positive rate* of the test. By simple arithmetic it can be shown that:

$$\text{false-positive rate} = [1 - \text{specificity}]$$

viz.

$$\text{false-positive rate} = b/(b + d)$$
$$\text{specificity} = d/(b + d)$$
$$(b + d)/(b + d) = 1$$
$$b/(b + d) + d/(b + d) = 1$$
$$b/(b + d) = 1 - d/(b + d)$$

$$\text{false-positive rate} = 1 - \text{specificity}.$$

Table 25.3 Verbal translations of kappa scores

Kappa value	Descriptor
0.8–1.0	Very good
0.6–0.8	Good
0.4–0.6	Moderate
0.2–0.4	Slight
0.0–0.2	Poor

Table 25.4 A contingency table from which the validity of a diagnostic test can be derived

Diagnostic test	Criterion standard	
	Positive	Negative
Positive	a	b
Negative	c	d

Upon finding the result of a test to be positive, practitioners should not assume that the result is truly positive. The result might be false-positive. Just how good a test is depends on the balance between the true-positive rate and the false-positive rate. This is reflected by a third statistic known as the *positive likelihood ratio*.

Conceptually, the positive likelihood ratio (+LR) is defined as the true-positive rate discounted by the false-positive rate, i.e.:

+LR = true-positive rate/false-positive rate.

Numerically it becomes:

+LR = sensitivity/[1 – specificity].

The utility and power of the likelihood ratio emerges from the following considerations.

If diagnostic confidence is defined as the chances of a diagnosis being correct, then it transpires that diagnostic confidence is a function of two factors: the prevalence of the condition being diagnosed, and the power of the diagnostic test being used to detect it, i.e.:

diagnostic confidence = function (prevalence; diagnostic test).

Because of certain mathematical idiosyncrasies, this relationship becomes complicated if diagnostic confidence and prevalence are expressed as percentages. However, it becomes very simple if diagnostic confidence and prevalence are both expressed as odds. In that event, it can be shown[2,4] that:

diagnostic confidence = (prevalence) × (positive likelihood ratio).

In verbal terms, this equation states that: the odds that the diagnosis is correct is the product of the odds that the condition is present and the positive likelihood ratio of the test used to detect it.

This equation underscores an important realization: that *diagnostic confidence is not dependent solely on the result of the test; it is also determined by how common the condition is.* Thus, for example, if the prevalence of a condition is 80%, the odds in favor of it being present are 80:20; and without applying any diagnostic test a practitioner can be 80% certain that the condition will be present. If the prevalence is only 10%, the odds in favor of the condition being present are only 10:90, and without applying any diagnostic test a practitioner can be only 10% confident that the condition will be present.

For a diagnostic test to be worthwhile, it must have the ability to increase substantially the diagnostic confidence based on prevalence alone. In this regard, the equation reveals what value the likelihood ratio

of the test must have in order for the test to be worthwhile.

If the likelihood ratio is only 1.0, the diagnostic test has no value. The diagnostic confidence is no greater than that which was available on the basis of prevalence alone. Just how large the likelihood ratio should be depends on the prevalence of the condition in question and how confident the practitioner wants to be.

Thus, if the prevalence of a condition is 40%, and the practitioner wants to be 80% certain in their diagnosis, the required likelihood ratio can be calculated as follows:

Prevalence = 40%
Prevalence odds = 40:60
Desired confidence = 80%
Desired confidence odds = 80:20
Diagnostic confidence = (prevalence) × (positive likelihood ratio)
80:20 = 40:60 × LR
LR = 80/20 × 60/40
= 6

If the prevalence is 10%, and the practitioner wants to be 80% certain in their diagnosis, the likelihood ratio is calculated as:

Prevalence = 10%
Prevalence odds = 10:90
Desired confidence = 80%
Desired confidence odds = 80:20
Diagnostic confidence = (prevalence) × (positive likelihood ratio)
80:20 = 10:90 × LR
LR = 80/20 × 90/10
= 36

If, in the preceding example, the desired diagnostic confidence is 90%, the required likelihood ratio becomes 81.

These examples illustrate that the desired likelihood ratio is not a singular figure; it depends on the context. The less common the condition, the larger must be the likelihood ratio; and the greater the desired confidence, the larger must be the likelihood ratio.

Conversely, consider how little diagnostic value tests provide if their likelihood ratio is small. If the prevalence of a condition is 40%, and the likelihood ratio is 1.2, the diagnostic confidence is:

Diagnostic confidence = 40:60 × 1.2
= 48:60
If expressed as a percentage,
48:60 = 48/(48 + 60)
= 48/108
= 44%

Such a likelihood ratio increases the diagnostic confidence by a meager 4%. Even if the likelihood ratio is increased to 1.5, the diagnostic confidence rises only to 50%.

These examples indicate that diagnostic tests with small likelihood ratios (i.e. close to 1.0) confer little change to diagnostic confidence. In other words, diagnostic tests with small likelihood ratios do not work well enough to improve diagnostic confidence to a worthwhile extent.

A corollary of these properties is that if the positive likelihood ratio is less than 1.0, the test actually decreases diagnostic confidence to less than what it was on the basis of prevalence alone.

ODDS RATIO

The odds ratio (OR) is a statistic that is sometimes used by investigators to describe data in a contingency table that relates two variables (Table 25.5). In such a table, if there is a relationship between the two variables, the values in the a and d cells should be greater than the values in the b and c cells. The odds ratio seeks to reveal this difference.

Explicitly:

$$\text{odds ratio} = ad/bc = (a/b)/(c/d) = (a/c)/(d/b).$$

In one sense, the odds ratio describes the "balance" between the two rows. It describes the extent to which the ratio of a as to b is greater than the ratio of c as to d. Similarly it describes the "balance" between the columns. It describes the extent to which the ratio of a as to c is greater than the ratio of d as to b. In another sense, it describes the balance between the two diagonals. It describes how much the product of a and d is greater than the product of b and c. Each of these interpretations reflects by how much the a and d values are greater than the b and c values. The greater the "imbalance" between these values, the stronger is the putative relationship between the two variables.

Historically, odds ratios have been used in epidemiological studies to determine the strength of association between exposure to a risk factor for a disease and the subsequent development of that disease. However, it is quite legitimate to use the odds ratio to compare other variables, such as two clinical signs, or the outcomes of two different treatments.

An odds ratio greater than 1.0 indicates that there is some relationship between the two variables; and the greater the odds ratio the stronger the relationship. Alone, however, the odds ratio does not indicate how clinically significant that relationship might be. In general, relationships start to become clinically significant when the odds ratio exceeds 3.0. Values greater than 1.0 but less than 3.0 reflect a definite but only slight relationship.

Odds ratios can also be less than 1.0. Such values indicate the likelihood of an outcome *not* occurring. These values can be interpreted qualitatively by taking the reciprocal of the value. For example, the reciprocal of 0.83 is 1.2. Thus, an odds ratio of 0.83 for an outcome not occurring is as powerful as an odds ratio of 1.2 that the outcome will occur. Accordingly, If an odds ratio of 3.0 indicates a strong positive relationship, an odds ratio of less than 0.33 indicates a strong negative relationship. Odds ratios between 0.33 and 1.0 may be statistically significant, but they do not reflect a strong clinical significance.

Mathematically, it can be shown that the odds ratio (OR) is related to the likelihood ratio (LR). Thus:

$$OR = ad/bc$$
$$LR = [a/(a + c)]/[b/(b + d)]$$
$$= (a/b)[(b + d)/(a + c)]$$

If we let d be some multiple of b, and a be some multiple of c, i.e.

if $b = md$
and $a = kc$
then,
$$LR = (a/b)[(md + d)/(kc + c)]$$
$$= (a/b)[d(m + 1)/c(k + 1)]$$
$$= (a/b)(d/c)[(m + 1)/(k + 1)]$$
$$= ad/bc(m + 1)/(k + 1)$$
$$= OR\ (m + 1)/(k + 1)$$

Thus, whenever, a is greater than c, and d is greater than b, the odds ratio will be greater than the likelihood ratio.

The advantage of the likelihood ratio, however, is that it is directly related to prevalence and diagnostic confidence, and so can be used to compute diagnostic confidence directly (as described above). The odds ratio could be used to the same effect, but would need to be reduced by the coefficient $(m + 1)/(k + 1)$ in order to obtain the correct arithmetic result.

Table 25.5 A contingency table from which the odds ratio can be calculated

Variable one	Variable two	
	Present	Absent
Present	a	b
Absent	c	d

REFERENCES

1. Cohen J. A coefficient of agreement for nominal scales. Educ Psych Meas 1960; 20: 37–46.
2. Sackett DL, Haynes RB, Guyatt GH, Tugwell P. Clinical Epidemiology: A Basic Science for Clinical Medicine, 2nd edn. Little, Brown and Co., Boston, 1991: 119–139.
3. Bogduk N. Truth in musculoskeletal medicine. II. Truth in diagnosis: reliability. Australas Musculoskelet Med 1998; 3: 21–23.
4. Bogduk N. Truth in musculoskeletal medicine. Truth in diagnosis: validity. Australas Musculoskelet Med 1999; 4: 32–39.

Index